Dancing with Cancer

(and how I learnt a few new steps)

Dancing with Cancer

(and how I learnt a few new steps)

Diana Brueton

Winchester, UK
Washington, USA

First published by O-Books, 2014
O-Books is an imprint of John Hunt Publishing Ltd., Laurel House, Station Approach,
Alresford, Hants, SO24 9JH, UK
office1@jhpbooks.net
www.johnhuntpublishing.com

For distributor details and how to order please visit the 'Ordering' section on our website.

ISBN: 978 1 78279 217 8

A CIP catalogue record for this book is available from the British Library.

Design: Lee Nash

Printed and bound by CPI Group (UK) Ltd, Croydon, CR0 4YY

To Chetan, Liz and Nigel.
To all my friends and relatives, medical practitioners, and those I may never know who have helped me along the way.
To Osho and Sogyal Rinpoche.

At the still point, there the dance is,
But neither arrest nor movement. And do not call it fixity,
Where past and future are gathered. Neither movement from nor towards,
Neither ascent nor decline. Except for the point, the still point,
There would be no dance, and there is only the dance.
– Four Quartets: TS Eliot

Introduction

You may not really want to read this book. An enjoyable read could involve a character going through all sorts of difficulties, but at least the reader can usually expect a clear and even happy ending. The story of a diagnosis of cancer can offer no such guarantees.

I'd love to have you with me in this journey though, and perhaps such a tale relates to us all, whether touched by cancer or not. Even when we immerse ourselves in the fullness and busyness of life, each day takes us closer to our own mortality. So we are all just a bit curious about how people cope with a diagnosis of serious illness. We wonder what our own reaction would be; we have a sense of pity for ourselves and others that life can be so challenging, and we strive to find meaning when life seems cruel and random.

That's why I'm writing this. It's to try to make some shape, some meaning, out of the time following my diagnosis of 'terminal' cancer. It's partly to let out the cry of 'not yet', but also to marvel at some of the extraordinary things that have happened, and to give thanks for life and love. I hope that's there's plenty of joy in it too.

Above all I hope that looking back on what has happened since my diagnosis, and seeing what still makes me so glad to be alive, may be of use to anyone else.

I have included extracts from journals I kept, a few quotes from teachers and writers who have given me sustenance, and some reflections that happened in the course of writing this.

I am told that in Buddhism illness is called 'the heavenly messenger'. May it be so. May I hear the message.

Thank you for being with me.

Chapter 1

It wasn't supposed to be like this. Midsummer in Cornwall held a promise of long sunny days, swimming, perhaps wobbling on a surfboard, above all idling on magnificent beaches. Unfortunately sitting on a beach had been a rare event so far in our holiday, as mists and rain made it feel more like autumn than the height of summer.

Finally a good day had arrived, skies had cleared and my partner Chetan and I were at long last on one of our favourite beaches. Here, where the wild Atlantic waves sweep over the white sands, crash against granite rocks, swirl in and out of rock pools twice a day, I have always felt my spirits soar.

So finding myself sobbing uncontrollably was a surprise. But here I was, feeling like my heart would break, and having no idea why. All I could say to Chetan was that I felt there was 'something black' inside me, and that I wished I could spit it out of me, let it be carried away by the incoming tide that swirled around the barnacle-covered rocks we sat on.

I put this sense of something dark within me down to letting go of the normal responsibilities of work and everyday life, and got on with the holiday. I did recall a drawing I'd done not long before, which looked really washed out, apart from a few black dots which speckled the faint, washed-out pastel. I had felt so tired when I did it. I just hoped the holiday would restore me.

After the sobbing on the beach, for a few days I would occasionally glimpse this dark black thing within me. We were staying in our little caravan perched high above the Atlantic. Occasionally the delight of being in Cornwall together would be momentarily eclipsed by the memory of those sobs. I thought it must just be something that needed time to process, that this holiday would help, or that it would reveal itself in time. Which it did, about six weeks later.

Perhaps this 'black something' was the first real sign of having colon cancer. There was certainly very little else to suggest it, just a slight feeling of more pressure in the bowel than usual, of needing to go to the loo a bit more urgently. Nothing to really alarm, to make me think it was anything other than, perhaps, a touch of middle-aged haemorrhoids.

I was actually much more preoccupied with a recent diagnosis of osteoporosis. That certainly did sound middle-aged. Could this really be me? I was 'only' 55, and dire warnings of crumbling spines, of hips that could shatter like glass, seemed extraordinary. Me? But I'd always been so fit. After never seeing my GP from one year to the next, I'd recently had to visit her several times to take on board this diagnosis. I had once or twice mentioned – almost as I left her – that something felt a bit odd in my bowels. But there had never been enough time to discuss it, until on one visit she asked more, and to my surprise referred me for a colonoscopy. Just to check it was haemorrhoids, she reassured me, and if it was they would probably 'deal with them' there and then.

So that was life before the life that was to come upon me, upon us. Chetan and I had been living in the middle of Dartmoor for some years. He earned his living as a self-employed woodworker, me as an art therapist. Living in such a remote place did present problems in finding and travelling to work, but for me this was far outweighed by being in this wild and beautiful place. Having lived in many places before, including Bristol and London, I didn't want to work all my life for the great day when I could retire to a place I loved – I wanted to do work I found fulfilling *and* be in that place. The wisdom of even this apparent certainty was to be questioned in times to come.

Meanwhile, life was good. A loving relationship, interesting work, a house, supportive relatives, friends, good neighbours. Work though was becoming more difficult, as cuts to NHS expenditure were putting a question mark over part of it. I had also worked for 13 years at Bristol Cancer Help Centre (now

Penny Brohn Cancer Care) and had finished there mainly because of the travel. But I had recently started setting up art therapy at a local hospice, work I had wanted to do for a long time, and hoped that work and finances would soon pick up again.

Going for a colonoscopy seemed a bit over the top. I even postponed it for a few days, so that I didn't miss a day's work at the hospice, which seemed much more important. Ironically, the pre-test concoction I had to take the day before the procedure was on a hospice day. I hadn't realised it would be so powerful, and had to go home early anyway.

Next day, August 10th 2007, a day now forever imprinted on my very being, I sat on a bench in the garden before leaving for the hospital and the test. A lovely sunny day, insects buzzing in and out of golden fennel flowers. I realised I wasn't enjoying the drink I was 'allowed' before the test. Perhaps I was a bit anxious after all, or maybe it was just the effects of the purging concoction. Taking medicines of any kind was something I always tried to avoid.

> Why write this, revisit the difficult past when the present is so precious? Outside, frogs are croaking loudly, the storm has awakened them. Maybe I too need to sing my song.

In the hospital car park I saw one of the chaplains from the hospice. We exchanged surprised greetings at seeing each other here. Gerry told me that he also worked at the Force Centre, a charitable support centre for people with cancer in the grounds of the hospital. I told him I was here for a test, but didn't say for what. I barely knew him, and 'colonoscopy' sounded embarrassingly like something that affected the elderly, not me – 'only 55'.

Did I really think I was immune?

So even as I headed unknowingly towards the precipice, loving hands such as Gerry's were already there to hold me. And they always have been – probably more than I will ever know.

The other patients were indeed elderly, and mostly men. Some waited with their wives and I wondered what they could be facing. I chatted with a nurse, talking about my own work in a psychiatric unit in the NHS. I was part of *her* world, not the world of old men staring into their possible demise, the loss of all that was known, was loved and familiar.

> Looking out to sea. Deep Mediterranean blue, azure. Will I live long enough to write this? Joy as I watch Chetan swimming, people enjoying the warmth of the sun on their miraculous bodies.

Suddenly I am in a different world. A world where I am no longer therapist but patient, no longer the strong but the weak, the sentenced. The one whose life has just screamed to a halt in front of a gaping abyss.

The doctor who had carried out the colonoscopy, leaving me in a pleasant, sedative-induced stupor, has waited for Chetan to come to pick me up. I am the last left on the ward, on a late Friday afternoon. Now he stands in front of me. He tells me I have a large mass where the rectum meets the sigmoid colon, and that in his experience it is almost certainly cancerous. And it has probably been there a long time. My body leaps involuntarily out of the chair, rigid. I have to face this standing up; it is impossible to remain seated. I have to look directly into his face. To face him, this.

The doctor explains what the likely treatment will be. Am I even remotely taking this in? I'm aware of standing as upright as I can, my back to the hospital bed, the dreary bedside curtains, this man at whom I stare intently, trying to take in every word as though one of them may contain a glimmer of this being a big mistake. There is no such word; he is very clear in his diagnosis. 'Ninety-nine per cent likely to be cancer.'

Chetan is beside me. Thank God.

I just about take in that I am to have a CT scan soon to see if there are secondaries, and following that the treatment is likely to be an operation to remove the affected part of the colon.

Late Friday afternoon. We leave the hospital along with staff hurrying to get home for a summer weekend. I am numb. At least on the surface.

Driving slowly through the rush hour traffic I see an overweight man walking along the street smoking. Maybe he is on his way to the pub, to home, wherever. How come his life is okay, while mine has just fallen apart?

That night we sleep fitfully. I manage to doze off for a while, only to wake with a terrific jolt at regular intervals as someone screams in my ear, 'You have cancer.' We cry, we hold each other. Will sleep ever be possible again?

I was certainly in shock, and probably remained so for weeks or even months at some level. My memory of the events that followed are sometimes vague and incomplete because of this, but some things remain razor-sharp. Above all the fear, the need to hold and be held by my friends and family, the sense of having been plucked out of the life I knew. And guilt – for what I was doing to Chetan, to everyone else whose lives would never be quite the same again.

By some good fortune we had invited friends for lunch on Sunday. So that gave Saturday a focus. We could cook, prepare food together, cry, talk.

First though I had to tell my family. I couldn't face it when we got home from the hospital, but knew I couldn't put it off. I sat on the edge of the bed with the phone, staring at the wall. I longed to be doing anything instead of being about to bring them such news.

My mother, my brother, my sister. All so loving, so shocked. Just the hardest thing, telling them. Wanting to reassure them, that I'd get through this somehow, and needing and receiving their love and care. Guilt. How would my widowed 85 year old mother cope with the news? My older brother would be upset, but wonderfully practical and supportive. My sister, 11 years younger than me, the one I should be protecting, how could I tell her? I now needed her protection. I don't know whether I was just trying to reassure her, or myself, or whether it came from a deeper place within me, but I said to her, 'Liz, I want you to know that *whatever happens to me* some part of me will *always* be all right.' I think we both knew I was talking about dying.

We made good food for Sunday's lunch. Chetan created a huge heart-shaped dish from an oddly-shaped marrow which he stuffed with vegetarian goodies. It was a tiny symbol of hope – or at least need – amidst the pain. We have been vegetarian for years (though when I hit the menopause I needed to add occasional fish), which added to the battery of questions that assaulted me. I'd eaten such good food for years, and I knew that colon cancer can be connected to diet. So why did I have this? This was a question which would come back again and again. It was a question that could torture, but which would also present me with more profound searches.

Was it diet, had I not taken enough exercise, drunk too much wine, inherited it, held on to emotions, eaten too many cakes, got it from living in a radon-rich place… just been unlucky? These questions would of course keep resurfacing, and do have their place in looking at what, if anything, needs to change. But for that day it was overwhelmingly just why?

The sense of disbelief was overwhelming, compounded by being virtually symptom-free. Perhaps a little more tired than usual, but no pain or discomfort. Colon cancer was the last thing I'd imagined getting. Breast cancer had always seemed much more likely, having quite a few of the potential contributory factors such as being childless. But colon cancer… vegetarian, no family history, relatively young, reasonably active. Yet I never doubted the hospital doctor's diagnosis even before the biopsy had been done; I knew he must be right. It didn't seem to be a question of 'why me?' but of 'why *not* me?' I thought of all those who had never had the amount or quality of life I'd had, who had died in infancy, been disabled for life, died unexpectedly or in war, suffered in many ways. I sent prayers to them, and gave thanks for all I'd had in my life. Perhaps it was now my time to experience what so many have known throughout their lives.

The friends coming for Sunday lunch had also worked at Bristol Cancer Help Centre. The timing was incredible. Could it be that some part of me knew they would be exactly the people I would need to be with at this time? If it was just coincidence, then many more such 'coincidences' were to happen, which have helped support me, maybe even kept me alive. I can only marvel and give thanks.

I broke the news of the diagnosis to them as they arrived. I was surrounded by loving arms, expert knowledge, practical help and a feeling of being totally understood in what I was facing. Helen, Thea, Ruth, Lisa and Hugh sat with Chetan and me in the sunny garden, all in a state of disbelief. We shared food, the heart-shaped marrow at the centre of the table, we shared shock, pain, friendship. Their work as therapists at BCHC has given them all a vast experience of cancer and what people with it go through, and to this they have each brought their own insights and expertise. I was to draw on that frequently, from each of them at different times.

We sat together until the shadows started lengthening. Before they left we stood together in a circle, arms around each other's waists. Someone suggested we 'tune in' to sending/receiving healing for me at 7 every evening. I was very moved that they would all be thinking of me each day, sending support. It seemed like such a lot to ask – let alone expect – from anyone. Yet another lesson was starting: how to receive, how to accept love without feeling unworthy. Perhaps the ego feels safer being the giver. Receiving is a much more vulnerable state. For me it instantly raised all sorts of questions about believing I was loved.

Before the circle ends I have a strong need to say something. I say to them all, 'I vow to live', with great force. I need that to be witnessed. Later I paint the words on canvas, and hang it where I can see it from my bed. Am I whistling in the wind? It doesn't much matter – it is also a statement that no matter how much time I have I still intend to *live* it. When I can.

> I scoop insects from the surface of the swimming pool, those that have not sunk to the bottom. Some dead, some alive, their translucent wings fluttering again. Some even fly back into the water – do they know the danger? I have lived in so much fear in my life. Do I dare to hope, or at least trust in life this day?

During lunch we had talked about what my treatment would be. I knew very little about what would be offered, just the probable operation after a CT scan, and that a specialist support nurse would be in touch with me. Having worked with thousands of people with cancer at BCHC, all of us are only too aware of some of the difficulties, and limitations, of treatments, and of the many 'alternative' treatments that have been tried over the years. Some of these have been hailed by their fans as cures; many more are part of the integrated medicine approach, providing physical, emotional and spiritual support alongside 'conventional' treatments. I would need to look at all these, choose what felt right for me.

I prayed that above all the CT scan would show no spread of the cancer beyond the colon. That was bad enough – but to have to deal with metastases... Such an ugly word, such an ugly condition. I had seen enough of what these could do – and even what they could look like if the tumours were large enough to show through the skin – to know this was definitely not a good thing.

And having secondaries implied chemotherapy. If I'd ever let my mind stray into 'what I'd do if I ever had cancer' territory, I'd always been adamant I wouldn't have chemo. Such damage it did to the body, awful side effects, surely there were better ways. My certainties about many things were soon to be challenged big-time.

The new week began. And it was new in so many ways. I waited to hear when the scan would be. Then there was work. I had been told the operation was likely to be very soon, possibly the following week, so all of a sudden I was having to tell my colleagues, and close down therapy sessions for the time being. Until, that was, I had recovered from the colon op and could return to work.

I left my NHS work with mixed feelings. I had worked in two of the units for many years, running art therapy sessions for older people with mental health issues. I loved the work, but recently new structures (inevitably to do with money) had come in, making the whole future of such groups unsure. I seemed to be forever fighting my corner for providing a service which I knew could be of great help to people. But the work took time; it wasn't like popping a pill and seeing instant changes. I wondered if it would still be possible to set it up again when I returned, or what would have happened by then.

The staff were concerned, kind and supportive as I said goodbye. One took the trouble to phone me later to tell me of her own colon operation, which was incredibly helpful. Someone I knew had got through this. My patients, to whom I just said I had a health problem, were kindly and a little bemused at my sudden departure. I felt I was letting them down.

Driving into Rowcroft Hospice, my other place of work, I thought as I often had of what it must be like for someone coming there as a patient. Would this be their last journey, or would they come back down this lovely tree-lined avenue again one day? And would I myself one day follow this same road, but this time as a patient? Possibly even to die. Melodramatic? Maybe, but such thoughts were inevitably there.

I arranged to come in to the hospice again before the likely op. I had only been there for six months, setting up art therapy. It was work I had long wished to do, and I was only partway through a trial period at the end of which its efficacy would be reviewed. I hoped it would then become a permanent part of the hospice's services. Little chance of that now, I thought, although in fact I was to be proved wrong later.

Bumping into Gerry on the day of the colonoscopy – just before the world changed – had been a godsend, maybe literally. On my last day at Rowcroft we met in the old wooden chapel that was home to music therapy and art therapy. He helped me make a bit of sense of some of the endless thoughts and questions that were bombarding me, to organise a 'filing system' of my mind a bit. But above all he gave me space – in my workplace of all settings – to start letting out some of the fear that I felt would overwhelm me. The fear was of pain and suffering, but mostly of loss, of death. Here was someone whose everyday life and work involved death and dying, who could address it without me feeling I had to protect him from anything, and who talked about it in respect of his own life and faith.

We sat in the old chapel, in the little 'sanctuary' I had been starting to create. It was painful to leave my work here, even if it was just for a while, as I thought. Thankful too to be able to start bringing these deep fears into the open.

I returned home, wondering when I might be back at work again, and thinking of what I faced between now and then. I wondered too how all those closest to me were coping, worrying about them, feeling guilty, but above all so very thankful that Chetan, my family and friends were just there. I felt they were holding me up, that without them I would fall to the floor, helpless. Which is actually what I did do not long after.

Meanwhile, I had a date for the CT scan. And my sister Liz was coming down for a few days.

Chapter 2

I walk up the steep single-track road that winds its way across open moorland. The twists and turns, the rocks and views are all familiar. The only things that change much are the sheep and ponies that graze nearby, and the colours of the gorse and heather. I have often walked up here to surprise Chetan as he returns home from work. If I have timed it right, I will have walked a mile or two in evening sunlight before I see him coming. I delight in the walk, and then in seeing him. Sometimes we stop on the way back together, walk along the stream and see the wild flag irises in bloom. We drive home chatting about the day's events. Our two cats greet us as we arrive, anxious for food and attention.

Now I go up the hill to meet Liz. A very different walk. I want her to know that I am all right, at least all right enough to do this. That I haven't slumped to the floor yet. I see her car in the distance, across the moor, and as she gets closer the look of surprise on her face as she spots me. It is so very good to see her. In the back of her car are trays of winter pansies, spring bulbs, pots and compost. We will plant them together, she tells me, a sign that there *will* be a spring to come. Perhaps she doesn't say it in so many words, but we both know the message, the optimism she wants to bring, even though I also know her fear and anguish.

Chetan is so pleased to see her too. I feel the goodness of us all being together. Lots of crying, lots of hugging.

The support nurse from the hospital had been in touch and Liz and I had decided to go in to see her together. Joan, the nurse, was available to answer our questions, she said, and guide us through what was likely to happen.

The weather had got a bit cooler. I needed a jacket, but didn't really want to wear my nice new one, for it to be 'tainted' by being in the hospital. But I wore it anyway. How many more chances would I have to do so? Such thoughts were never far away, and even if I dismissed them as 'ridiculous' did they not contain a grain of truth too?

The last place I wanted to go back to was the hospital, but of course the place of such distress also offered the hope of help. Joan explained to Liz and me about the four stages in which cancers are categorised, ranging from 1 to 4 according to degree of containment or spread. She felt sure mine would be 'only a 1', and would be operated on to remove it. She showed us the ward where I would be a patient – not bad, I thought, at least it was quite light and bright.

Talking about how I was right then, I mentioned I was slightly constipated. Joan looked a bit alarmed and started talking about 'obstruction' in the bowel, and what might help. In fact I think it was the shock that seized my body up, and made my bowels determined not to let go of anything. Joan suggested I buy some Movicol, a laxative.

All of a sudden I seemed to jump from someone who almost never took any form of medication to a person saying yes to all manner of chemical and man-made concoctions. Instead of saying no thanks, I think I'll see what effect psyllium husks, prunes, syrup of figs etc have, I just *had* to get some Movicol. We toured Exeter town centre looking, not as we normally would have done for clothes and treats, but for a powerful laxative.

Which I never took.

We had talked with Joan about the CT scan, which would be in a few days. There seemed to be all sorts of provisos about dates of seeing people afterwards, because of team meetings, holidays and so on. I could not bear the thought of other people knowing the results for days on end before they could see me in person, so I asked Joan if I could be informed of the results as soon as possible. A mistake.

Liz and I went for lunch, usually a joyous occasion. I just couldn't eat much, and felt so bad as Liz had paid for it. Had I turned from a healthy, fit person with a good appetite to someone with cancer just picking at their food in only a few days? Again, I think it was the shock, but it was certainly also a reminder that my body was not as I thought I knew it to be.

Liz's visit gave both Chetan and me a much-needed boost. Her warmth and vitality lifted us, and seeing her and Chetan caring for each other, even laughing and joking at times, reassured me too. Daily news of her husband Paul, and two boys Joe and Tom, was a reminder that there was still life beyond what was happening to us.

> The beachside bars have closed for the season. Storms come. But the bar-owners have given up too soon. We walk barefoot along the seashore under cloudless skies.

It's Friday afternoon, two weeks almost to the hour since I was told I probably have cancer, now confirmed by the biopsy. Another sunny day, but a world away from that day, my life now full of trembling and trepidation. Waiting for news of the scan is awful. The phone rings, but it must be too late in the day to hear anything.

It's Joan, calling from the hospital. A strange time to ring, so late on a Friday. She sounds reluctant to talk – is she edging around the subject, putting it off? She can't avoid it any longer.

I have secondaries in the liver.

I fall to the kitchen floor. It cannot be true. I kneel, grovel on the ground, a chair is just not enough to contain me. Please let the floor swallow me up, too. I vaguely take it in that Joan will be in touch next week about seeing the surgeon, but that it may now put the colon op in doubt. At least, I think that's what she says.

Then she is gone. I'm hysterical, gasping for breath.

Liver secondaries? To me that only means one thing. Incurable. Death. Probably fairly soon.

I was alone in the house; Chetan would probably not be back

for some hours. I grabbed the phone again. Just before Joan had phoned I was speaking with an old friend, Fran. She and her husband Jonathan were due to come the next day for the weekend. I called her. She was the perfect person, and I owe her a debt beyond words for being there, in every sense of the phrase. She must have been utterly shocked, but miraculously found exactly the right words. I sobbed down the phone to her about dying, how I felt I had had a good life, that I was terrified, that I didn't want to die, and above all how on earth I was going to tell Chetan. Fran somehow made me feel that from many miles away strong arms were holding me as I fell apart.

Chetan was right in the middle of moving his carpentry workshop. He was just finishing taking all his gear from the old place to a new one. I didn't even know if I could get hold of him, as mobile phone reception on Dartmoor is erratic. I could not bear the thought of bringing this pain to him.

Fran and I agreed that she and Jonathan would still come the next day. Again it seemed that amidst the trauma life was supporting us. Jonathan and Chetan are old friends from university, and I had come to know and love them too. If they could bear to come, I knew it would be the most immense help to us.

Meanwhile I managed to locate Chetan. I'm not sure if I was more relieved or aghast when he did answer his mobile. He was just taking out the final load. I asked him if he could come home, right now. I didn't tell him what had happened, but he set off at once. I cannot imagine what his 12-mile drive back was like.

Fran had suggested that I take some paints out to the garden while I waited for him. For me that's a great way of letting things out. I grabbed sheets of paper and in the garden hurled paints at them. I dug into the paper ferociously, scribbling 'how can I tell my beloved Chetan?', crying, hysterical.

All I now remember of him coming home is going to meet him and walking up the path behind him. Green trees in the garden, early evening light, the back of his neck. Knowing that I had to tell him this news when we got into the house.

> A boy swimming in the sea is in difficulty. Everyone rushes to help, a lifeguard dives in. The boy is all right. How connected we all are. I too have known the kindness of strangers.

Jonathan and Fran's visit is a godsend. They arrive with wonderful food and staunch friendship. We are cosseted and cared for.

Ruth, who had been at the Sunday lunch that first weekend, called in too. She had already been coming by, phoning, a tower of strength. Her knowledge of cancer, both medical and emotional, is deep. Fran, Ruth and I sat in the garden together. To either side of me was a caring, strong, practical and sensitive woman whom I needed very much.

I still haven't told my family, more than a day after hearing about the metastases. I just can't bear it. I can't put it off any longer. Fran sits with me. I need her strength. Telling them is agonising, I wonder how they will bear it. Going into the hospital with Liz had made everything more real, more possible to cope with. But this is a whole new scenario, one with a far worse prognosis.

I feel a bit shivery at times. Must be the shock. Fran wraps me in a blanket. Their whole visit leaves us feeling wrapped up in love and reassurance, even though it all feels so terrifying.

Next day was August bank holiday. I was in pain, quite bad. What was happening? Was I obstructing, as Joan had called it? I had severe pain in my side and my abdomen. No GP service as it was bank holiday, so we had to go to the local hospital to see the on-duty doctor. I had been there several times two years before, when I had broken my ankle and a bone in the foot. Waiting forlornly to see the doctor I wondered if that event, which had been fairly traumatic, had anything to do with this condition. If there was any one common thread I had seen in people at BCHC with cancer, it was that many of them had had some significant episode or period of stress a couple of years or so before the cancer. Yet another factor to wonder over.

The doctor was kind and caring. I had a temperature, and he diagnosed diverticulitis, an inflammation in the colon. It was probably caused by the CT scan, he thought, and I was sure the last two days must have been a contributory factor too. I was prescribed antibiotics, and took them gratefully. I was fine in two days, but it had been another intimation that my body was not as I had thought, that difficult things were already happening. I had even quite expected to be sent to hospital, sure I was obstructing… scary new scenarios were rising unbidden.

Recovering from the diverticulitis, there were other challenges. What treatment was I going to be offered? When would I see a consultant? Why did no one at the hospital seem to have taken into account that there was a bank holiday, meaning the usual multidisciplinary team meeting was *not* meeting and that any appointment would therefore be postponed for a week?

> We travel through Spanish mountains. Arid and rocky, scarred by mining. I want to be somewhere else. I struggle to accept where I am, what is.

Ruth visited again. She brought flower remedies for us both, to help with the shock. She also brought her reassuring presence, and her experience. Joan had been in touch with me about a meeting with the surgeon, Miss Boorman. As we talked this over with Ruth we started seriously wondering why I was still being referred to a surgeon. It sounded as though surgery just wasn't going to be on offer, so why waste time seeing her? Ruth suggested querying this. I did so, only to be told that I was still officially the surgeon's patient, and the way ahead was through seeing her.

On one of Ruth's visits – all the more amazing as it was some distance to our remote house – she showed me how to do 'tapping', or emotional freedom technique (EFT). It helps to ease fears and anxieties, and replace them with something more positive, by tapping acupuncture points while repeating a particular phrase. I tapped in, 'Even though I feel fear and grief, the divine loves and supports me unconditionally. I am calm and peaceful.' It was useful to have that to turn to at times, as it engaged the mind as well as allowing emotions to rise up and then settle back.

Just letting go of that awful phone call was a work in itself, and one which will perhaps never quite be complete. Although I had asked Joan to let me know the scan results, perhaps a way could have been found for telling me in person, or at least making sure someone was with me when the gravity of the situation had become apparent. To be told that on the phone, alone at home, is traumatic.

I was recovering from the diverticulitis, and at last had a date to meet the surgeon. It had all taken so long from initial diagnosis to the surgeon's appointment. But at last there was some hope of getting a fuller picture and starting treatment.

Or so it seemed.

Chapter 3

The wall of love, Chetan called it. As friends heard of my diagnosis I received many cards, flowers and phone calls, each one a nugget of soul-food. As more cards arrived Chetan started putting some of them on a large pinboard. It would be a reminder of people's love every time I walked in the room, he said.

It wasn't just a reminder. It was a gradual allowing myself to believe that I was, am, loved. A theme I would return to.

I wondered if I myself had always been such a good friend. I certainly knew now the value of expressions of love.

As part of that support my cousin Martin and his wife Paddy had agreed to come to the consultation with the surgeon. Martin had recently retired as a consultant, Paddy is an ex-nurse, and I felt that having them there would be tremendous support. They would understand all sorts of things that I would not. I knew too from having met so many people with cancer that it can be hard to take in all that is said in a consultation, so their expertise would help immensely in that way too. Again, just the fact that they were prepared to come a long way to be there with us touched me greatly.

Some time later Martin sent me a newspaper clipping about research showing that people with cancer who have strong family support do the best. If that is so, I should live to be 100!

Chetan and I meet them at the hospital. Strange to be with them somewhere other than the more usual social family gathering. We discuss what we know so far – I realise surgery is going to be unlikely, but need to have this clarified and to know more.

If the day of the colonoscopy and the day of being told about the liver secondaries were awful, this was on the same scale. No, worse. It would drain me of hope. Even now writing about it is excruciating. Even now I need to have my hand held to endure it. Thank you for being with me, reader.

We are ushered not into a consultation room, but into a tiny examination or treatment room. It is windowless, with an examination table against one wall and two or three chairs. More chairs are brought into the already cramped space. Miss Boorman arrives, with Joan and another nurse. We are sitting almost knee to knee.

Miss Boorman, tall and athletic, greets us. I explain why Martin and Paddy are there, who they are and that they are here to support me. Her colleagues prop themselves against the door and wall; I am aware of them behind me but cannot see them, only Miss Boorman. It already feels intense.

She tells me that surgery is not possible. The reason, she says, is that there are many tumours in the liver, some large. Operating on the colon would be pointless as it is the liver that is the most threatening to my life.

And besides that, she says, I have cancer in the lymph and quite possibly in the lungs.

In the lungs? The lymph? My head falls forward onto my hands. If there had been any floor available I probably would have dropped onto it.

I am told by the surgeon to sit up, that I need to listen to what I am being told. Does she think I have dozed off in the back of the classroom? I am doing my best to bear it, to keep my mind engaged so that I can take it in, ask what I need to ask. I am so grateful Martin and Paddy are there with us. Chetan holds my hand; I cannot bear to look at him. Miss Boorman is good enough to show Martin the notes and discuss them with him. I am reeling, in complete shock.

I feel like a guilty prisoner. Surrounded by the surgeon's 'henchmen', I am being condemned. There is little feeling of kindness; this message must be delivered with headlights blazing and I am the terrified rabbit caught in them. Take this in. You are now sentenced.

I will, I am told, be referred to an oncologist for chemotherapy. They will be in touch with an appointment.

My memory of this meeting is of course subjective. I can only say that's how I experienced it.

Reeling out of the hospital, we needed to sit together, have a drink and talk. The Force Centre (at which I knew Gerry sometimes worked) was a haven, as it would be many times again. Its welcoming atmosphere allowed us to find a quiet corner, complete with tea and biscuits brought by kindly volunteers. Martin and Paddy explained a little more of what had been said. But the verdict was clear. No surgery. Chemotherapy.

They told me of a friend of theirs who had recently had a similar condition. Following chemo which shrank the tumours he had been able to have bowel surgery and was now well. Perhaps there was a glimmer of hope there for me.

But still… the lymph, the lungs. How long could I survive? I did not want to know.

Chetan, my beloved Chetan. What was I putting him through?

In the Force Centre we discussed the long delays there had been in getting even this far. Diagnosis upon diagnosis, but still no treatment. It looked as though I wasn't going to get to see the oncologist, Dr Osborne, for some time either. This just did not seem right. We managed to get hold of Dr Osborne's phone number. Chetan was surprised to find himself speaking to her in person, not to a secretary. She sounded kind and understanding, he said, and realised I would be wanting to get treatment going as soon as possible. An appointment was arranged, not too far off.

> Thousands of swifts flocking, swooping and swirling in the blazing sunset over the sea, preparing to fly down to Africa. I am humbled by their journey together.

At last one good thing. If having chemo is what you call good. I had always thought it was something to be avoided at all costs. I would have to give this real thought, consider all possibilities, be sure of what I was doing.

As we were about to leave the hospital, having thanked my cousins for going through this with us, we felt reluctant to go home. Perhaps being alone was too much straightaway, and the journey from the hospital to home is at least an hour. I phoned a friend who lives along the route, told her what had happened and asked if we could drop in. She was too busy, she said. This was very painful. But understanding and forgiving such events in my life would turn out to be an important part of what I have needed to look at and be with.

Lisa and Hugh, from that first Sunday lunch, also live on Dartmoor, and welcomed us in for tea as we drove home. We sat in their beautiful sunny, late summer garden. Their kindness and support were backed up by the best cucumber sandwiches I've ever had, eaten as we sat in their garden swing-seat. Just starting to take it in.

> Is this the last of summer? Ink-black skies obscure the mountains and sea, momentarily revealed by mile-high lightning. Deep thunder follows quickly. Maybe the storm will quieten and summer will last a little longer.

Much later, Chetan told me he thought Miss Boorman probably didn't expect me to live for more than six months. Actually, he told me that more than two years later.

Chapter 4

It is eight in the morning, fresh and bright beside the river. I am doing chi kung exercises on the banks of the East Dart, close to home. My neighbour Ines has been teaching me for a few days. She has given me a great gift. Chi kung seems so life-affirming right now, especially getting up early to do it in this lovely setting, and it will continue to be an important part of staying sane and well.

It is almost mid-September, and the gorse bushes are enmeshed in cobwebs covered in dew, reflecting dazzling low morning sun. It seems incredible, at this time of such desolation, that I feel so alive. As Ines and I perform the graceful movements (well, graceful in her case) and the river rushes over the boulders, I suddenly feel this is just what I've been wanting to do for a long time. I realise I have neglected making time for things like meditation, yoga, 'inner work' that nourishes me. I see the irony of only redressing the balance as I face a life-threatening condition, but I'm alive now, and this is what I need and want.

I started keeping a journal, which has continued to be a great form of release. I'm including extracts here (in this type).

Standing by the rushing river. Such bliss! The sun on my face, the water flowing and cleansing me, opening me up. I have wanted this for so long. Now I open up to life, to healing, to love.

I had met with Dr Osborne to discuss chemotherapy. I liked her, she was sympathetic and took time to explain things to me. She showed me the scans of my body, in particular of the liver where the large tumours could be clearly seen. Great black blobs. Really big ones in the right lobe, several smaller ones in the left. Seeing them there on the screen, not just being told about them, made it so much more real. How had I managed to live even this long with all that in me? I thought of the certainty I'd had on the beach that I had 'something black in me'. Now I could see it.

I told Dr Osborne that I did not want to know what my prognosis was. I felt that if I was told I would probably live a certain amount of time, when I reached it I would surely expect to die, like 'having the bones shaken' at you. I couldn't face knowing either. I needed time to accept that at 55 my life was no longer to be measured in decades, but in small numbers of years, or even months. I think, though, that if I had asked I may have been told to expect two years with the chemo, if I was lucky. I have been.

Chemo, if I decided to have it – and this was a big if – would be for three months, or according to what I could tolerate. It could, she told me, be stopped at any time if I found it too much. It would consist of an intravenous treatment every fortnight, for which I would come into hospital as a day patient, with a second drug taken orally at home most days in between.

I don't know what to do. Is there an alternative – other than a quick death – to this chemical onslaught? I know there are all sorts of diets and regimes that can help, but this is a drastic situation.

Ines tells me of the Oasis of Hope clinic in Mexico. She urges me to look into it before making a decision, which I do. I have heard of it before, and know that it has achieved good results and also emphasises spirituality and, of course, hope. But something doesn't feel right about going there. It's hard to say why, but it seems wrong to be running in desperation to a poor country when I haven't explored what is under my nose.

> News from England of glorious late September weather. Here it has deluged, all night and all morning. But regretting choices I have made takes me nowhere. Now clouds are thinning. People return cautiously to the beach.

I had to make a decision – to accept the chemo or not? I dreaded the thought of all the side effects, and wondered if it might ultimately do me more harm than good. I asked for guidance.

That night I dreamt of a big green road sign, with names of various destinations written in white on it. Most of the lettering was quite small, but written large in the middle was 'NHS'. I knew this meant I should go with what the NHS had to offer – in other words, chemotherapy.

But I also understood, even as I was dreaming of the sign, that NHS meant not just National Health Service but *healing* service. This was part of the message too. That it wasn't just about taking the chemo, it was about healing. I knew this could mean many things – doing all I could for my body, of course, but also healing on other, deeper levels. It was about whatever would support my body physically through the chemo, but it also meant the start of a journey, a process of healing. After all, the dream was of a road, with the sign just showing me the way along it. It is that road I'm still travelling along.

So chemo it was to be, but backed up by all I could do myself, and with the help of others. And other people were crucial. I craved to feel loved and supported, more than I had ever done in my life.

Realising I doubted that I was truly loved was to become a huge learning process for me. I felt unworthy, not good enough – an old story for lots of us. I am still learning that this is not just a question of the ego, but of discovering how connected we all truly are, that we are all part of a universal flow of energy. But even getting a glimmer of this would take time. Meanwhile I welcomed those cards coming in the post, the phone ringing with good wishes.

Before the chemo started Chetan and I met with the chemo ward matron for a rundown of what was to happen. For once it was a pleasant room. Comfortable chairs, windows and even the offer of a drink seemed to acknowledge the pain of the situation. I was given dire warnings of what to expect – possible nausea and vomiting, maybe hair loss though not as likely as for a hormonal cancer, burning hands and feet, mouth ulcers, lowered immunity and consequent risk of infections. I should be careful if gardening not to scratch myself because of this, to avoid emptying cat litter trays, and so on. I knew a lot of this before, but now it was not just knowledge. It was how I was going to live, what I might face. Despite the attempts to make it more human, it was scary stuff.

There were to be six chemo sessions in hospital, spread over 12 weeks. I drew up a rota of people who would come with me so that Chetan didn't have to come each time. This was also good for both of us in making us feel we weren't in it alone.

First on the list was Liz. The first chemo.

> A cicada skitters along the edge of the pool, dangerously close to falling in. Good, it has headed away from the water. Why do I care if it lives or dies? But I do.

Liz and I arrived at the hospital a bit early and went into the Force Centre for a bit of TLC and a drink. Chamomile tea in my case – I had given up tea and coffee as soon as I was diagnosed, to give the poor liver at least one less strain. A man sitting nearby heard us talking about the forthcoming chemo, and asked if he might tell me of his own experience. There's always a fear when someone says this, that you may hear something you don't want to hear, but he was clearly offering me support in a vulnerable moment. He told me the chemo he had had for lymphoma had not been too bad. He had heard my fears, and now told me he was in remission, if not cured. Even though it was a different cancer, and I knew that great strides had been made recently in chemo treatment of lymphomas, he gave me a real boost. He had seen my distress and reached out to me, as so many people have. It felt like a hopeful sign. It also taught me something about the kindness of strangers.

I walk into the chemo suite, as it is called. Seven or eight easy chairs are ranged around the wall. Each one has a metal stand beside it for holding fluid drips. I am invited to choose a seat, and Liz sits with me. The nurses are friendly, efficient. They have done this so many times, and it is a routine I too will soon come to know well.

A bowl of warm water is set in front of me as though for a ritual ablation. I steep my hands in it to help the veins appear, so that one may be chosen and pierced. I have already had an ECG to check that my heart was fit for chemo – something I would never have doubted before, but now I am unsure of anything about my body. And now, how will it take this invasion?

Anti-nausea, steroids, saline solution… various things are dripped into me, clearing the way for the chemo, Oxalyplatin. It has arrived, brought up from the pharmacy on a tray like a precious gift bearing my name. Liz and I hold hands.

In my other hand, the one now bearing a needle strapped into it, I hold a small red velvet heart embroidered with the words 'I love you'. My nephew Joe has given it to me. I would bring it with me to each chemo.

At last it is time for the chemo. I ask the nurse if I can write something on the bag of drugs. She looks surprised, but agrees. It is easiest for Liz to do this, given the status of my hand. 'The things I do for you!' she says, but bravely, in front of the nurses, writes on the bag 'Healing Love'. This is partly a wish, of course, an incantation to summon up all forces divine or earthly to be with me. But it's more than that too. Masaru Emoto's extensive research appears to show that the properties of liquids can be changed according to the thoughts directed to them. I am happy to try anything that may help, if it resonates with me.

The chemo starts to enter my body. Through headphones I listen to gentle, flowing music. To my surprise I don't feel fear that this concoction is entering my body.

What I feel is gratitude. Huge, huge thankfulness that I am receiving this. I think of all the people who have been part of creating this drug – the researchers, scientists, doctors, administrators. Their commitment has brought this to me. Letting myself go deeply into the sensation of what is happening, there is only vibrant silver-blue light, with plasma-like specks of gold and other colours dancing through it and going to all the cancer cells.

> It is nearly daybreak. One last frog sings after a nightlong chorus. I am fearful of the day, of the writing that lies ahead of me. But right now the frog has stopped, a bird sings, light is spreading.

We have brought food in with us, a lovely meal that Chetan has made. He would do this every time; it seems so important to be sustaining ourselves with good food. I am even able to eat with no difficulty. Liz goes off for coffee; I am alone, just me and the chemo. I feel okay. At the moment I rather avoid contact with the other patients, needing to keep my inner strength, fearful of being dragged down and fearful of 'negativity'. Later this will change, as it did with the man this morning. I will open up to sharing and the support we can give each other; but right now I just focus on my inner space, on what is happening.

Liz returns. The chemo has finished, just some flushes to be put through the vein and then it is all over. She has got me through it.

Arriving home, there is a huge bunch of flowers from Richard and Valerie, another cousin and his wife. What wonderful, sensitive timing.

Chetan looked so anxious when we got back, but between us we had made it. We hugged each other, all in it together. I needed to go to bed early, but was so happy to hear Liz and Chetan chatting, sharing some wine.

Next morning I started the oral chemo. I sat quietly, taking my time to swallow the tablets. This time the sensation was of fiery red coursing through me, burning all the cancer.

Part of the chemo support is steroids, taken to prevent nausea.

I was supposed to take steroid tablets for three or four days following the intravenous treatment. Unfortunately they also make you very energised in a wired-up way, and my sleep was quite disturbed. At first I didn't mind too much, I was just so relieved to be having treatment that I hoped would give me more life. But I knew that if I had too many sleepless nights it would be horrible. In time, as it became apparent that nausea was not a problem, the steroids were mercifully greatly reduced.

Sleep could be a problem, though, whether I was in a steroid phase or not. Hardly surprising. Fear in the middle of the night is a painful place, even with someone beside you. Even with all the support I was receiving, I knew it was my fear, my journey into illness, treatment, possible death, that I needed to address. As for us all, I must eventually face this alone.

I used all sorts of techniques to try to get back to sleep. I would work through my body from feet to head, tensing and relaxing all the muscles – gently, so as not to disturb Chetan. I would try to visualise myself in a beautiful relaxing place, like a warm sunny beach. One of the most effective ways was to visualise all the love that I knew was being sent my way surrounding me, like a cocoon of white or gold light. Sometimes it would change to purple, and would flow inside me too like a great flame.

And in the mornings – chi kung by the river, while the mornings were still light enough. It was wonderful to be able to do that even though I was on chemo. Ines would encourage me so much, countering my fears and 'what ifs' with 'Yes, but how are you now. Good?' and I would realise that in that moment I was fine.

A few days after starting chemo I dreamt of a great boulder being lifted out of my body by two angels. They threw the boulder into the sea, to be scoured and cleansed, then brushed me down with a white feather. Walking down to the river in the early morning I saw a small fluffy white feather. A little message? I laughed for being so fanciful, but when a rainbow appeared too I couldn't help reflecting that there are things around us which we are only privileged to glimpse from time to time. Perhaps this was so with the healing power of the universe. It would take me time to know that this could come in many different ways.

Chapter 5

Was the chemo doing any good? It would be impossible to tell for a while. It all seemed to hang on the CEA count, which shows the level of cancer activity. My count was around 6,000 – very high. The hope was to bring it down, as this would be an indication that the chemo was having some effect. There is of course no guarantee that chemo will do this, it doesn't always.

We settled into a kind of grisly routine of fortnightly trips to the hospital. I would be anxious about getting there on time, but the real anxiety was more profound. Seeing the consultant before the chemo was nerve-racking. If certain blood counts were too low the treatment might be refused this time, and now I was desperate to be able to have it.

Autumn became a time of letting go. I was letting go of my life as I had known it. No more work. No more control over so many things. My brain felt as though it had been zapped with a cattle prod; I was incapable of dealing with even everyday things like paying a bill or reading the post, let alone all the information I was being deluged with about cancer. Bit by bit Chetan took over much of this from me.

> Rain falls. I was not prepared for it. Just two more days of holiday. I am desperate for it not to end this way, for there to be more sun, more joy.

I had to sell my car. We couldn't afford it any longer, and we clearly weren't going to be needing two vehicles. Though it was a bit of a wrench – it was a nice car and part of my independence – it was after all just a car. And it brought a huge benefit, as the buyer was an acupuncturist who I have been seeing ever since. His treatment has supported me greatly, at times quite dramatically, transforming a sleeping or eating problem literally overnight and always boosting the healthy, flowing part of my energy.

Another autumnal letting go was of any pretence of being completely in charge of my life, capable and independent. All of those beliefs – had they always been an illusion anyway? – were being chipped away at.

My brother Nigel and his wife Judi brought my mother to visit. It was difficult to know if Mother really understood the seriousness of my condition. Aged 85, it seemed cruel to burden her with that, but I was unsure if her staunch positivity was real or a defence. But whatever it was, it was how she was dealing with it, and I felt so awful that she should have to. I cried in the kitchen with Nigel and Judi. Later we all walked along the river. I put my arm around Nigel. He has been a tower of strength and support.

Autumn half-term came, and Liz booked a holiday cottage by the sea to which I was invited. Chetan stayed at home to have a bit of time to himself. Suddenly there was sea and beach walks, and all my angst being wondrously counterbalanced by young boys hanging off the stairs, digging massive holes on the beach, joking, eating pizzas. Sometimes I would feel so separate – I couldn't bear to even see the ridiculous skeletons when the boys watched *Pirates of the Caribbean*. I knelt beside the bed at night praying. But it was a dose of young life, salt air and above all love.

The chemo started taking its toll. I got more exhausted, and as time went on would find myself suddenly drained, usually tearful, and would need just to go to bed for a while. But I didn't feel sick, though over time my appetite lessened and I found many foods unpalatable. Baby-type foods, like mashed potato and scrambled eggs, became my favourites.

I wanted to explore all possibilities for treatment and support, ranging from the orthodox to the way-out.

Dr Rosy Daniel was one of my first contacts. She was medical director at BCHC while I was there, now working privately. With a huge range of experience, Rosy is truly an 'integrated medicine' practitioner. She thought I was doing the right thing with having chemo, as I needed to 'staunch the flow'. Not only was this reassuring, but Rosy also gave me lots more contacts. I did not know at that time that her later suggestions would, I believe, save my life.

I gathered information from many sources, such as Cancer Options and Cancer Support. I investigated supplements, treatments such as being encased in a sauna-like box, oxygen therapy, diets of cottage cheese and linseed oil, adrenalin therapy, visualisation, 'natural' chemotherapies. Rosy stressed that there were more treatments available for the liver than what she called the 'bog standard regional oncology' usually offered. This would need looking into. Meanwhile, just having all these other options to at least investigate gave me a feeling of hope, that there was more I could try which would help right now and after chemo.

We have the house dowsed for negative energies. Is it my imagination, or does it feel more flowing and sparkly afterwards? I want to do all I can to let in healing, vibrant energy. A dowser tells me to visualise angels putting a huge rose quartz under the house, to change the geopathic energy. 'All is frequency,' she says. I place a rose quartz under the corners of the mattress, get rid of the electric blanket which seems to emit static, and tune into feelings of love, emanating it to every cell in the body. She talks of the power of prayer, suggesting I say 'I do want to move forward, I do want to live.'

This dowser also told me of Silent Unity, a Christian organisation based on the idea that all is already perfect, we just have to find that connection within us. They offer a phone prayer service, open to anyone, which I found really supportive. There were times when I needed to be reminded that I was still valued, still seeking. Their booklet of daily prayers became part of my everyday routine. In the past I would probably have dismissed it; now it was a warm place to dive into every morning.

I dreamt I was going down a ski slope. It looked tricky, but to my surprise I found it quite easy, I had the ability to do it, and I could see I was going to make it on to the flat section ahead. I am coping, I feel ok right now, I need to remember I have the ability to cope and that I am doing so. I was even enjoying the downhill skiing.

I gradually built up a regime which I'm sure helped me through the chemo. I'm including it here in case it's of use to anyone, but stress these were just my personal choices.

- Vitamins D and K (supportive of chemotherapy)
- Slippery elm regularly, to aid the digestive system, including putting a paste of it in the mouth last thing at night, to help prevent mouth ulcers
- Psyllium husks to aid digestion
- Salvestrols
- Zeolites
- A good mouthwash – not chlorhexidine as this destroys 'good' bacteria too, and a soft toothbrush to prevent mouth damage
- Colloidal silver to protect from infections
- Vitamin C only in moderation, as it can interfere with chemo uptake
- Pau d'arco tea, soothing for the stomach
- Dandelion coffee, liver-cleansing
- Quercetin
- Curcumin
- Milk thistle
- No yeast in food if possible, to stave off thrush from chemo
- An acid-free diet if possible
- Omega oil
- Linseed oil
- Iscador (a homeopathic remedy – I asked for a referral through my GP)

- Selenium
- Magnesium citrate
- No caffeine
- Fresh vegetable juices
- High calorie build-up drinks (not from a packet)
- Maitake tablets
- Acidophilus
- Homeopathic remedies
- Organic food
- Something to eat in the night to keep the calories up
- Castor oil body packs
- Soothing teas such as chamomile
- Regularly moisturising feet and hands as chemo makes them very dry.

Most of this was just to support the physical body. I knew that my thoughts and inner being needed even more attention. And this is what my time with cancer has been all about. Pat Pilkington, co-founder of BCHC, uses the 'Hero's journey' of myth as an archetype or metaphor for the cancer experience:

> *The Hero leaves all that is familiar, comfortable and companionable, and in the dark before dawn, rises alone and sets off to journey to the far country. It takes consummate courage and faith to face the 'dragon Fear' and rescue the 'Maiden': the true Self. The Hero returns, changed by the experience.*

I certainly doubted my courage and faith, and was becoming quite intimate with the 'dragon Fear', but I knew it was the search for what Pat calls the 'true Self' that I needed to embark on.

I evolved a first-thing-in-the-morning routine, before I got up. It helped to set me up for the day to spend time in prayer, doing a visualisation, centring myself into the earth, praying for my loved ones to be held and cared for.

I tried meditating. Chetan and I have been sannyasins, followers of the Indian meditation teacher Osho, for many years, yet for a long time after the diagnosis I just couldn't meditate. My body seemed incapable of sitting or lying still; it just wanted to jump up, not give itself up to letting go into whatever ghastly scenarios the mind might present. It took time for meditation to return.

Lots of anger, fear. Anger at just not *wanting* this, and fear of what may lie ahead. Yet right now I am fine, just find it difficult when I get tired, weepy, wobbly. What helps when I get like that? Sometimes to let it out very forcefully - scream, shout, cry. Sometimes resting, finding a peaceful inner space.

Many other things helped me through that difficult time, and still do. Receiving healing became incredibly important. The 'laying on of hands' calmed me, brought me into myself without it being too terrifying. Chetan gave me healing sessions almost daily, before he became really exhausted and needed to stop. I would sometimes feel the presence of other beings with us, and would enter a peaceful, dozy space, at times seeing lights and moving energies. On several occasions I sensed Chetan's grandmother with us – she had been a nurse and died of bowel cancer. It was a precious way for us to connect beyond words, and always took me to a more peaceful state. Helen, who had been with us that first Sunday after the diagnosis, came to give me healing too, and those times would become very important. If I was on a Hero's journey (as indeed we all are) I certainly had and have the most extraordinary companions.

Another neighbour, Michelle, brought me CDs of Louise Hay. I lay in bed listening to inspiring encouragement to love and respect myself, to let go of blame of others and myself, to forgive, to live joyfully – all of which she sees as essential to healing.

'Positive thinking' can sound trite and patronising, but Louise Hay has herself had cancer, and recovered from it. I found her words uplifting. Even if this approach did no good physically – though I sensed it did – I needed to feel I had some control over my life, my feelings, my thoughts, maybe too my illness. I would often listen early on a sleepless morning before going to the hospital for another round of chemo.

> I slip into the pool just a little less cautiously than the first time. Sun glints from the waves I make. My scarred body is less fearful. My body. I am still in it.

Another wonderful neighbour, Carrie, gave me kinesiology sessions. It seems to tap into the body's 'truth', going beyond the conscious mind to see what it needs, and giving help through meridians and energy fields. It always put me into a more energised, positive place.

In one session I told Carrie I had an ongoing, anxiety-ridden dream of not knowing what I was meant to be studying at college – what the syllabus was. We came up with a new 'syllabus'. This one was quite unlike anything academic. True, there was finding out more about the goddess, but there was also connecting with the seasonal rites and rituals, dancing, music – lots of much juicier things.

I dreamt of 'hopeless' and 'hope' being weighed in the balance on a set of scales. When I put a pearl on the 'hope' side it became much heavier and outweighed the other side. I was told the pearl was the pearl of wisdom, to do with self-knowledge, and that this was what would tip the balance.

I also used, and use, visualisation. The power of the mind is great, and using it to direct healing towards the cancer again gave me a sense of some control. Besides which, I think it helps. I would relax my body, imagining myself in a beautiful place, then direct a great wave through my body, seeing it as sweeping in a great tide of healing energy and all the nutrients I needed. As the wave broke on a beach I would see foamy water engulfing each cancer cell, which would be powerless to resist, and die. More water would then wash the residue from my body. This changed with time, and I later also visualised DNA cells changing.

Lisa gave me craniosacral sessions – very subtle and beautiful. Someone described craniosacral as 'being meditated'.

Early in the chemo process we were visited at home by our GP, who brought with her a nurse from Hospice at Home. That title really knocked me – they obviously thought I was dying. But actually that visit turned out to be a great gift. I saw how much our GP was doing for us, and the Hospice at Home nurses have been fantastic. One of our biggest difficulties at that time was finances, and they steered us through the tangle of claiming benefits. They later provided some complementary therapy sessions at home, and more than anything have been there giving practical and emotional support.

Had my fourth intravenous chemo yesterday, so am now into the second half of the six-chemo cycle, if that's what will happen.

Hardly know how to begin writing about how it's been so far - so many losses, much fear, mercifully no pain, increasing tiredness which has been very hard to accept, but I'm now getting more used to trying to go along with it - even to enjoy when possible!

I need to find a 'new skin', one that protects me, lets in the good. It means being a bit like a chrysalis, growing a protective new skin whilst doing inner work, not setting agendas, having expectations of myself, just resting in myself, allowing that space until the time comes to emerge into finding new purpose in this wonderful world.

One morning we received a phone call to say that some tests Chetan had recently had indicated he needed a prostate biopsy.

We both felt shattered. How could we cope with this too? But that was just the start of that day. The same morning brought news that one of his sisters had a brain tumour which looked very serious, and then that a child of friends had attempted suicide. I felt as though a sledgehammer was dealing me blow after blow, hammering me into the ground. It just seemed unbelievable, but was sadly true. By great fortune I had already scheduled a kinesiology session later that day. I came out of it feeling as though the hammer had been lifted, that although this was all awful stuff it hadn't yet completely flattened me. The attempted suicide, we heard later, had thankfully survived. We could only pray for how the other two situations would resolve themselves.

Chapter 6

Living in a glass box. That's what having chemo is like. I could see life going on all around me, people going about their normal business as though they would live forever. 'Normal' for me now was feeling more and more tired, spending a lot of time resting in bed. I could be doing something very ordinary, taking it for granted, when the un-ordinariness of it all would suddenly hit me. It was as though I had indeed walked into a glass wall, had smacked up against the realisation that nothing was the same any more. That I was probably dying. Maybe quite soon.

But I still went to every chemo session reciting to myself, 'Chemo is my loving healer. It destroys all cancer in my body, and nothing else. I am healthy, fit, happy and healed.' And I gave my body that message first thing every morning.

My body has suddenly become quite strange and alien to me, as though it's not really mine. Will it suddenly get an infection from some small thing it would previously have shrugged off, what's this tiny ache I would previously have ignored? So... it's time to befriend it. To own it. And in particular to acknowledge it for the fantastic job it's done all my life, and still now. Thank you, lovely body. Let me know what you need. I'll love you, not be scared of you.

Occasionally I saw Gerry while I was having chemo. It was always reassuring, knowing that he had this great depth of experience and understanding of illness and death. He also told me of his personal experiences of bereavement, and his certainty that his loved ones were literally still there with him. I found this more difficult to accept, though yearned to. On other hospital visits we would sometimes visit Exeter Cathedral. Its sacred space was still and holding, a gift from our predecessors. We lit candles, and asked for prayers for healing.

I went to Bristol for a homeopathic consultation. Amazingly, there's an NHS homeopathic hospital there. I wanted to be prescribed iscador, a homeopathic treatment derived from mistletoe which is purported to help with cancer, and support chemotherapy. It's used extensively on the continent, but is relatively unknown here. I obtained some thorough research that has been done into its efficacy, and my GP referred me to Bristol.

The homeopathic hospital is just up the road from where I was born and spent the first nine years of my life in Bristol. I need to go and look at the house. I have been having flashbacks to being there as a child, feeling frightened at night in what feels like a huge, dark room, and knowing there is a great black hole of a cellar beneath me. It is strange to be at the hospital, so close to that early part of my life, the streets so familiar. I visit the house which I haven't seen for many years. I could see that a large Victorian house could be intimidating for a small child – its big windows look exposed, it doesn't seem cosy and inviting. Yet it was a great house too, with big rooms and a garden where Dad built a swing in the old apple tree and a sandpit. So I imagine myself as that little girl back then. I tell her she is safe and loved.

We stay with Janet, a healer at Penny Brohn Cancer Care. I feel welcomed into a loving family house, accepted. Janet gives me a healing session. I feel the pain and sadness of when I stopped working at the Cancer Help Centre, of no longer being part of something I'd felt so drawn to be part of. It is bonfire night, and I can hear fireworks going off outside. They become part of the healing – explosions of light going through me, strong and strengthening.

A magnificent sunset spreads across the sky, over a calm sea. Bats flit across it and the moon is almost full. No wonder we sit late after supper, watching in awe. Tomorrow we return home.

I visit my mother, who lives close to Bristol. It is painful – I can see her pain so clearly, and know there is little I can do about it, other than reassure her I will be all right. Which is indeed the truth at some level. I try to use my time there as an opportunity to release some of the difficult feelings I have about our relationship. I ask the two angels from my dream to lift what feels like a rock in my guts of guilt, anger at myself, pain at having not been able to connect with Mother as well as I would have liked. I ask them to help me release this. My poor mother, having to cope with so much now. I can feel how excruciating it is for her.

I can't relax and let things happen, they might fall apart. What's behind that? Fear. Of things falling apart. Of not being supported. Of not being *worthy* of support. That's been instilled in me, and I feel rage about having always had to 'earn' being worthy. Yet remember, just a few minutes ago Chetan had his arms around me and said 'let me take care of you.' Why is that so difficult?

Before the diagnosis Chetan and I had booked to go on a Deep Memory Process Workshop in November. Deep Memory is about accessing past lives. We had done a couple of these workshops before, and I had found them extraordinary. They had convinced me that we do indeed live many times, and that these past lives can have lessons for us in our present one. Perhaps above all they showed me that life is far more than we experience in this brief span we call our life, that our consciousness is endless. While religions teach us of life after death, some even of reincarnation, these workshops had made theory a reality for me. So I was desperately keen to be able to do this workshop, to explore further and also to meet up with old friends from the workshops. I just hoped I would be well enough.

Luckily the workshop didn't clash with a hospital treatment. We travelled to north Devon, me letting the window down every so often to let in a blast of winter air. The chemo was giving me hot flushes – different from menopausal ones (I'm now an expert on hot flushes). They would start with a strange feeling in the solar plexus and within seconds I would be drenched in sweat.

The first night of the workshop. We sit together, perhaps a score of us, in a circle in a cosy bar. We are actually sitting on a circular bench and around a beautiful round table which Chetan made. I am so proud of his wonderful craftsmanship. I look at the faces, recalling work we have done together reliving past lives, past deaths. It has a different, more urgent aspect for me now. Taking it in turns to talk of what has happened since we last met, I wonder if I will be able to talk without crying. They all look so shocked as I explain I have cancer, it's inoperable, I'm on chemo.

I wake early next morning from a vivid dream or vision. In it a gigantic woman rages like Kali, bestriding a river on which I am being borne along, guided by other women. It is terrifying to pass beneath her, through her massive bare limbs, but even as she rages to the skies I know that she is also protecting me and that this journey along the river is part of my healing.

The workshop is intense. I find myself in a past life where I was a woman cast out of society by religious bigots for bearing an illegitimate child, forced to live on the margins and eventually killed brutally. This seems to be the pattern of many past lives I have encountered. Perhaps there are lessons I'm living out in this lifetime, about my own rage, about forgiveness and maintaining hope of how life can be, of regaining the real equality of men and women and true spirituality.

I rage and rage in the workshop. Roger and his assistant, Jen, support me completely in screaming, shouting, thumping cushions in an urgency to expel this disease from my body. To allow in healing and love. I drink in the wisdom of Roger's teaching, and the love I am given by my fellow time-travellers.

Jen became a huge support for us, visiting us at home. She would come with gifts of wonderful books to share, especially about goddess religions. I thirsted to know about the ancient veneration of the goddess, in history and as she reveals herself in our lives now. I needed to find that part in myself. To acknowledge the raging, raving, dancing, nurturing, soft, powerful, creative and destructive female energy. I saw signs of her all around me – in the fecund tor shapes on the moor, in the flowing river. Reconnecting with a power that has been suppressed for so long in our world was acknowledging what needed to be changed in myself too.

> A heron takes off from beside the river, its sculpted shape prehistoric. We are back home on Dartmoor. Herons are said, in China, to be lucky. The heron comes back again.

A scan in November. Fear before it, but the news was good. The tumours were shrinking. Chemo was having an effect – the CEA counts were 'moving in the right direction' as the consultant told me. Fran, Liz and Lisa each came with me to sessions, giving Chetan a break and me a real boost each time. I knew that decisions would have to be made. My three months of chemo would finish at Christmas. What would happen then?

Yet still the consultant was talking in terms of 'adding months' to my life. I wanted years.

Awake early from the steroids. Tired, went to bed early but kept waking from a deep sleep. I felt as though I had journeyed into some deep, dark place - a place of all sorts of fears I would not wish to be with, darkness. I had to pull myself out of it each time, to carry on sleeping, only to awake again, trying to climb back up, to see myself in the light. I try to stay in the present, in the light, surrounded by love even though that's hard.

We were starting to research other possible treatments for when chemo finished. I visited a doctor who specialises in 'alternative' chemo treatments. It was painful, seeming to reinforce the seriousness of the situation, that surgery would probably never be possible. I faced the fear that despite the good scan, nothing would really help, and I would either succumb to a passing illness or decline into distressing effects of the cancer.

While a miracle may happen, it may not. I move between acceptance, fear, grief, trust, love, despair. I ask for grace.

A beautiful day. Sannyasin friends visit, we meditate, sing, eat the lovely food they have brought. We talk about fear, and each one gives me a little nugget of helpfulness:

Atosh: 'It's impossible to stay in meditation when the fear just sweeps through you. Anchor yourself through the senses – hear a bird singing, look at nature, to bring you back.'

Nisheetha: 'Go deep into the fear, looking at what's within it, the different layers. Ask the fear "who are you?", going more and more into it. And seeing death as a great mystery.'

Luci: 'See the fear as a small child, imagine cradling it in your arms, loving it, cherishing it.'

Fear was indeed the issue. A huge ball of it in my solar plexus, almost physically sore, like a wound. In a healing session with Helen she helped me approach it, to release some of the blackness there, bring light to it.

Chetan and I decided to visit a famous psychic surgeon, Stephen Turoff. He is renowned for the healing work he does with people, sometimes producing physical signs of his work on the body. I certainly wasn't sceptical, but neither was I expecting a miracle. I just felt that any healing input could only be of benefit.

Stephen's clinic is in a little Portakabin behind a motel in Chelmsford. A most unlikely setting, and Stephen turned out to be a most unlikely healer and mystic. Dressed in bright orange Indian robes, he is a giant of a man with a strong Cockney accent, so robust and energetic for someone working with these mysterious energies. I lay on a couch, and he placed his hands over my abdomen. I could feel nothing other than the soft pressure of his hands, and cotton wool being wiped across my skin. As he worked he talked about fear. He certainly knew where I was at! He spoke of his childhood, during which he had suffered severe illness and had apparently died twice. 'It's not dying that's difficult,' he told me, 'it's living.' He quoted from the Bible, spoke of our journey on Earth, and of living fully each moment. It might be a cliché, he said, but you could be knocked down tomorrow by a bus, so why not live fully now.

As we left the clinic we crossed over the busy dual carriageway, on a pedestrian crossing controlled by lights. Out of nowhere a car came hurtling along, clearly didn't see the lights and was within a whisper of knocking us down. Yes, I thought, I get the message, Stephen. Anything can happen at any time. I'm still struggling to live in the moment, in joy and trust, but I know that living consciously is what it's about.

Later that day I found what looked like scars on my abdomen – over the colon and the liver. I had not felt anything at all that could have produced such marks.

Christmas was approaching. A very different one. I couldn't go shopping, and longed to give people something to show my love, this Christmas and in times to come, when I might no longer be here. Even shopping on the Internet was exhausting, but I did it, hoping I had bought gifts which would have some meaning – silver pendant for Liz, spiritual books and a cuddly cashmere jumper for Chetan.

Liz has invited us for Christmas with her, husband Paul and boys Joe and Tom. I wake to the day with a sense of both joy and anguish. So many Christmases. Will this be my last one? I am thoroughly spoiled and cosseted all day.

Christmas Day, still in bed, feeling good. Yesterday was difficult, a lot of grief - being here, Christmas, the boys. But today I feel filled with love. I know I am loved. I am so thankful and grateful. Why be sad, It's about now.

It was good too to see Chetan having a rest. I could see he was getting very tired from all he too had been going through. He was also concerned about his sister, soon to have a major operation, which she thankfully came through well.

Christmas also marked the completion of three months of chemo, which was the initial duration of treatment. But I'd gradually come to understand that I could have double that amount if I felt up to it. And I did. Apart from exhaustion and some loss of appetite I was fine, and determined to carry on as long as I could. I felt the chemo was helping, and it was.

New Year's Day 2008. Yesterday went for chemo number 8 and discovered that my tumour blood markers have come down a lot. I just feel so good. I know huge things lie ahead, but I'm going the right way at the moment. I welcome 2008 as a time of living fully and joyfully.

We saw in the New Year with Fran and Jonathan, a time for celebration, for being beautifully cared for, for giving thanks for all they had shared with us in the last few months. For being alive.

Chapter 7

The new year had started with good results but I was possibly only halfway through the chemo. I wanted to be able to do the full twelve cycles, which would take me up to the end of March, but had no idea if I could manage it.

I'm tempted to not write about the rest of the chemo. There was exhaustion. There was the constant regime of medication. Lack of appetite meant that mashed potatoes, bananas and other 'nursery' foods were top of a limited menu. Finances became a big issue, and would become even more pressing. The question of what would happen after the end of chemo was always hanging over us. I could see Chetan becoming increasingly exhausted as he had to do more and more for me. But there were good, uplifting things too, which helped me then and encourage me now in writing this.

I tried to develop this 'good' within me. Every morning while still in bed I went through a process of relaxation, prayer, and visualising the body as whole and healthy. I needed to find a stillness, a place within me that was completely healthy whatever my body was doing. I tried to accept healer Barbara Ann Brennan's words, 'Be still and know that I am God', not in an egocentric way but to find the divine within, to strengthen myself in knowing that.

> Raking up fallen leaves in warm October sunshine. Another year of doing it. What was once a chore is now a pleasure.

Perhaps the decision to get married was part of that. I wanted to mark and celebrate the love Chetan and I had shared for many years, and also thought it might make anything to do with hospitals easier practically and, to be blunt, with officialdom should I die. Chetan graciously accepted this, even though marriage was something he'd always regarded as state intervention. We planned to marry at the end of March, as soon as I had finished chemo. I had a wonderful time ahead to plan for.

I dreamt I was in a city by myself. Just this great feeling of loneliness, aloneness. Later I spoke with Janet, who said it's so important to have lots of support at this point in the chemo, to feel I can let go into that. She and the others in Bristol are sending me healing, which feels so reassuring. She added that as I recover from the chemo I can find a new way ahead, my own creativity, to use for *me*. But right now to rest, and especially to feel the support.

If one of the big lessons of life is letting go, then this was a crash course in it. A small thing could suddenly hit me. One time it was a memory of Chetan and I driving down to Cornwall with the caravan, carefree and excited. There was a well of grief in me for what might never be again.

In a healing session with Helen I feel that grief like a black lump in my solar plexus. Slowly, slowly, it releases, my body seeming to extend, stretched by bands of brilliant colours that surround me. Helen and I rejoice in sharing these mysterious experiences. Later, in bed, I see the most intense, dazzling lights over me and all through me and give thanks for whatever is happening.

And sometimes I just needed to watch an old movie, to chat to friends, to think of anything other than 'my condition'.

I started writing down things that I'd read which inspired me, and that I could dive into again at times of need:

The feminine mystery lives now.
Its energies are concentrated
on what is happening in this moment:
the scent of wet pine,
a hesitant hand.

The feminine does not save itself
for some glorious moment
in the past.
It holds nothing back,
Now is all there is.
– Marion Woodman

The honouring of 'the feminine mystery' seemed part of what I needed to acknowledge within me. I had been too caught up in all the doing, competing, proving myself aspects of life. I'd no idea whether that had anything to do with my illness, I just knew that in order for me to feel more complete in my life, in what was left of it, I wanted to find a new balance.

On the moors near where we live there are many ancient remains from our distant ancestors – hut circles, standing stone circles, burial chambers. Lying in bed one day I recalled a visit to two circles of standing stones near us. Close together, one seemed to have feminine connections – maybe a burial site – and the other male, but they seemed quite cut off from each other. I promised myself that as soon as I could I would visit the circles and find some way of linking them together. I also decided that I would climb the nearby Bellever Tor, one of the highest points on Dartmoor.

I would make that journey, I decided, at the end of chemo. If I could.

> A perfect October day, all is golden and blue. From the train window I see people on the little Devon beaches sitting in warm autumn sun beside a calm sea. I am on my way to London for a scan, trying to stay just in this day.

I talked to my body. I asked it what messages it had for me. 'Live courageously,' said my liver, 'live fully.' The bowel spoke of clean, new energy, of letting go – as it should, of course, but now in a more profound sense. The lymph looked for vibrancy, movement and light bringing in a new way of life, and the lungs told me to have the courage to expand. It was all about letting go of my previous life, moving into a new one.

Which sounds great, but isn't so easy in practice. One day Chetan felt unwell too, and even one of the cats fell ill. It all felt too much, dragging ourselves around trying to cope just with existing.

Next day we both felt a bit better, and Fred the cat looked happier too. It had been so hard the day before to believe life would ever feel any better again.

And so the two-week cycles of chemo continued. Sleeping poorly the night before, anxious about arriving on time. Sitting in a run-down, windowless waiting room to see Dr Osborne, scared of what she might tell me from the blood test I had to have each time before the chemo. Then sitting in the chemo waiting room, fastidiously trying not to touch much in case I picked up an infection, staring at the fish tank they'd presumably put in to calm us, waiting for my name to be called by one of the kindly nurses. Then, after all the needles, the dripping in of bags of chemicals, going home with relief but wondering whether the steroids would mean I slept little that night.

Staying at Liz's for a few days after chemo yesterday - number 10! Liz, Paul and the boys looking after me so beautifully. The tumour markers yesterday were down to 794!!! Amazing, after 5000+ in November. Thank you for the healing.

Saying thank you for healing was also an attempt to let my body know this is what was needed, and what was happening. And of course I was overjoyed that my body clearly was responding to the chemo.

The time at Liz's was wonderful. I'd initially felt a bit nervous about leaving my little cocoon of support with Chetan and home, but it was a precious time. One evening Joe, knowing I wouldn't drink alcohol, made me a herb tea complete with tiny parasol and fruit on the edge, just like a cocktail.

Back home, a new venture started which has continued to give me great support. I went to a Native American medicine wheel course, run by my neighbour Carrie. I was rapidly coming to realise that I have extraordinary and gifted neighbours. I was so excited to be there – that I felt well enough to cope with it, but above all to be embarking on a new spiritual experience. I have found the wisdom of the medicine wheel to be extremely profound, honouring as it does all aspects of our selves and the world, integrating us into a greater vision of life. At times that first day it was a little scary, venturing into this new world, but so rich. There was a sense of adventure.

Can it really be so far into January? Time feels quite strange at the moment - things that happened just a few days ago feel eons away, and at the same time as though time has stood still. Perhaps It's a mixture of the chemo and these grey, damp January days that are still very dark. Yet there's something beautiful about this time too. A sense of hibernation from the dark dreariness, which reflects my own need to cocoon myself in relaxation and healing.

One day I see daffodil shoots in the garden, and a few snowdrops peeping through. The promise of lighter days, of regeneration, resonates within me. Doing the medicine wheel has made me feel I can explore new areas of myself and my connection with the world. It has also given me back a sense of belonging, that I *am* part of the whole, not isolated as some strange being by going through something that separates me from others.

I really enjoyed doing some clearing in the garden. New shoots were coming through under the old dead leaves. Being in the sun was like a kiss on my face. So many blessings - Ines, so full of energy and support, kinesiology with Carrie letting go of ancient hurts. Dearest Liz who phones me nearly every day. I am in awe at the many blessings in my life.

I could veer within minutes between acceptance and deep grief. I cried a lot, particularly at certain parts of the chemo cycle. I dreamt of being with other art therapists, and realised I would probably never do that work any more.

Lot of sadness. Yes, a lot of sadness. Best not to try to cover that up, but to acknowledge and accept it. Sadness at no longer being part of art therapy work. After meditating, I had a vision of an owl. It took me into a very dark wood, to where it lived. I felt I was being shown that even the very darkest place has some light, that it is also home, that there is nothing to fear if you look correctly.

There was pain too for how weak I must have been prior to the diagnosis, but had struggled to work thinking it was just some resistance. I cried when I remembered one day when I'd felt I hardly had the strength to drive to work, to do the session, but had still done so. I cried for myself, realising that now I had to learn how to care for and truly love myself.

Trying to get clues for what might help me in this crisis, I looked back at one of the most difficult times in my life. What had got me through then had been discovering meditation, and becoming a sannyasin of Osho. I was able to do a little more meditation bit by bit. One morning I woke with an intense feeling of Osho being with me, a richness of him filling my third eye like a sun. I felt drenched in energy, gratitude and an intense sense of surrender.

I did some artwork from time to time, always finding it very emotional. But it was a struggle, my energy was so depleted.

The owl appeared to me again in a kind of vision, sitting high up in a dark tree in a forest. It knew the darkness was fearful for me, and reassured me it would be alongside me.

I'm letting the tears come. Sometimes it's very emotional, other times I sob in a very physical, almost un-emotional way. I wonder if this is about letting go of things I've absorbed and which my body now wants to rid itself of. Releasing the pain and shock too. Sometimes I wake in the night and just feel the sobs there within me. It's so good to trust that I can release them without getting hysterical or traumatised now.

Chapter 8

It's four in the morning. I'm in the kitchen, eating muesli. The cats are hoping they're in for a very early breakfast.

I'm feeling fine, despite the post-steroids wakefulness. I hear an owl calling, a sound I now find reassuring in the deepest dark of the night.

It's the middle of February, only a month or so until the chemo is finished. And then there may be other decisions to be made, about what to do next. Will I be able to have an operation? Will I need to look at other options?

Later that day the colorectal support nurse from the hospital phones me to discuss a recent scan. Hearing her voice is painful, instantly reminding me of the time she phoned to tell me of cancer in the liver. She tells me very clearly that surgery will probably never be possible, however much the tumours shrink. Although I knew that was already what they thought, it is very hard hearing her say that the cancer is so widespread in the liver that it precludes an operation. That is still their position. And the implication is that operating on the colon would be a waste of time because the liver would get me first anyway.

A small part of me never quite gives up, though, on the hope that maybe one day an operation may be possible. We've been trying to track down doctors who might have a different opinion, but while I'm still on chemo this is homework rather than actuality.

To calm me, Chetan gives me a healing session. I have a strong sense of a woman putting her hands gently around my chin, looking intently into my face and saying very clearly, 'There is nothing to be afraid of.' Chetan tells me later that he was 'instructed' to put his hands in just that position. I know it is to do with the work I have been doing with the goddess, invoking the divine female presence. This seems to be confirmed when I go into the bedroom. I've recently put a photo of Mother Meera, the 'divine mother' there and I feel my gaze held by her eyes for a long, long time as her face moves and shifts as though the photo is alive. It is very intense, very moving, like being mothered and held by the mother of all mothers.

Healing sessions weren't necessarily always blissful:

I found it difficult, struggling to let go, relax. Towards the end of the session a sensation of dense blackness going out of me, almost like toothpaste being squeezed from a tube. Intense, not easy. But afterwards, a brilliant white light shining on me as though from a many-faceted crystal.

We yearned for a break, perhaps somewhere with some winter sun. We even pored over travel brochures, looking for somewhere that also had spiritual connections. Maybe Malta, with its goddess sites. But what about travel insurance? What if I got ill? If it was a fantasy, which really it was until chemo was long finished, it was probably one we needed, a promise of escape from dark days.

> The weather has turned and the morning light comes later. I have had golden days of joy. Today I get news from the scan. I travel to London through glowing autumn countryside.

There was one thing we definitely could look forward to though. Our wedding would be just ten days after I had taken my last chemo tablet. It would be low-key, as my energy levels were so fragile. We hoped to then go to St Ives for a couple of weeks in the caravan. There was much joyful planning to be done, including buying a new dress. A rare treat. Shopping trips had become a thing of the past, but Internet shopping for a new dress was such a joy. I thought I'd better add a pair of shoes too!

Chetan went away for a night, the first time since I'd been ill. Although I felt particularly delicate as it was the day after an IV chemo treatment, all was well. Our neighbour Ali visited me, bearing soup and friendship. She has given us generous support and our friendship has grown – this illness seems to have provided space for these miracles. And learning to ask and receive has been a big lesson.

Nigel brought Mum to visit, which was also very touching. So painful, feeling that I had inflicted so much on them. I had learnt she had probably had a small stroke a couple of months ago, and could only feel I'd been at least part of the cause. Mum told me she had dreamt that I was in an operating theatre, that I got up from the table and walked towards the door, cured! I wondered whether this was her own wishful thinking, or whether she really did know something that I didn't. I told her what I'd been told about the impossibility of an operation, but she was quite adamant that this dream had something to it. Should I feel angry at her apparent covering up of reality, or delighted that she held this hope?

'This is the day that the Lord hath made: let us rejoice and be glad in it.' I bounce between fear and hope, grief, loss and joy in being alive. Yesterday I welled up with grief for all the lovely times Chet and I have had in the caravan. Yet they are in the past anyway, whether or not I'm ill.

As the end of chemo approached, it was a good time to start looking forward a bit at what I would like to have in my life. It felt vital that my 'wish list' was not going to pressurise me, to turn into another burden of achievement. So it included things like spending time with people I love, being by the sea, meditation, dance, being in nature, painting, cycling, making the house and garden lovely, visiting some inspiring places.

My hands and feet became sore and burning from the chemo. At its worst it became difficult to type on the computer, like having thick mittens on my hands. I gave up trying to get my emails correctly written, and hoped people would forgive me for the many typos. The feet were more difficult. It was like walking on a thick layer of broken up hot Maltesers. My feet would burn in bed at night, and walking any distance became difficult. But it was all manageable physically. I was never sick, and didn't lose my hair. Coping with the emotions was far more difficult for me. Sometimes I felt truly ashamed of that, thinking of what so many people have to endure. And the irony that despite having worked with so many people with cancer I was still finding it so hard to cope with myself. I felt very humble.

Reading something about cancer yesterday suddenly made me feel absolutely hopeless, that there is no way I can recover. I cried, cried, cried until my heart felt like it would burst. Such grief, utter helplessness. Chetan held me, I cried for ages. He said later that he knew it had always been difficult for me to be alive in a physical body, to feel safe - maybe because of all the past lives I've explored where my body was burned, abused, etc. That has been there all my life - fear, not honouring the body, wanting to 'space out' from the body. And I saw that in the crying and the helplessness there was still that idea - that it will all end in fear, pain, suffering, that there is no hope of recovery really.

Yet there was a huge part of me that really did still want to live. I usually woke in the morning with a feeling of great joy that another day had arrived. I decided to 'reprogramme' my despairing part. I drew myself standing on the top of Bellever Tor, arms raised to the sun. I told myself:

It is safe to be in my body
I love being alive
I wish to live for many more years
My body is healing
I love my body
I love being alive in this body.

Walking beside the river I would sing out loud, making up words like 'I rejoice to be alive.' I felt I was reconnecting to the land, and to myself.

I desperately needed that. When chemo stopped I would have to make decisions about any other treatment options. That was a scary prospect, trusting that I would make the right decision, and that I would know all the possibilities.

> On the train home. Late afternoon sun picks out sheep in green fields, seagulls against dark, ploughed earth. I need more treatment. I am tired.

But first I had to get through the last days of chemo. It was getting gruelling. Exhaustion, above all else. Trusting that I was healing, that it was working. Lots of painful dreams. Swinging between days of grief and utter tiredness to ones where I felt more energetic. Lovely healing sessions with Chetan that nearly always took me to a more peaceful place. And many painful dreams.

When I woke from a dream I felt that something in my body has decided it's too early to die. That there's lots more time before that, and to come 'home' and live a lot more first. That feels pretty good.

I truly did feel that something in me had decided to live a lot longer. I realised how much I love my life, and gave thanks for it. For perhaps the first time in my life I was starting to feel I could be my authentic self, that I could live in beauty, in this body now, in gratitude.

I was reminded of Osho's words:

> *This very body the Buddha, this very earth the lotus paradise.*

Chapter 9

Jen, Carrie and I are climbing the steep hill to Bellever Tor. The brilliant late-March sunshine holds a hint of spring, a gentle warmth. The grass is still parched and golden from winter frosts, but soon new green shoots will grow through.

It is the last day of chemotherapy. I have been so hoping to be able to climb the tor, to affirm that I have come through these six months, but have been worried that a cold I felt coming on might prevent me. But I have woken feeling that I can manage it.

In the night I was aware of a huge presence near me, amorphous, silvery. I didn't really want to look at it, but it kept being there. I realised it was death, which was why I didn't want to look.

Then it coalesced into a silvery-blue column of light, and was very definitely feminine, and soft and loving. Not remotely frightening. I felt 'she' had always been there, that I wasn't being shown this because death is imminent, but because I've been looking at this, needing to see it. And now I know there is nothing to fear. And now I continue to live.

We three women seem to be performing an ancient rite, processing to the top of the tor. I stand on the top, raise my arms to the heavens and to the expanse of Dartmoor laid out below me, remembering all the times I have spent in bed just imagining this. I hug the rock in gratitude. And tomorrow is spring equinox, with its promise of new beginnings.

When we come down from the tor Carrie holds a Native American pipe ceremony for my healing. She calls on Grandfather Sun, Grandmother Earth, the plants, the animals, the humans, the little people, the crystals of the earth, the planets, the stars. We pass the pipe around between us, and I ask for guidance to see the way ahead, to find peace, solace and healing.

And the way ahead is a little frightening. Reaching the end of chemo means no more hospital visits, no more monitoring until my next meeting with the consultant in a few weeks. All of that is great, but it's also a bit like having the stabilisers taken off the bike. I'm on my own for a bit now. Chemo goes on working for quite a while after treatment has stopped, so the consultation in a few weeks will show what effect there has been. It's not an appointment I'm relishing.

Meanwhile, just before the walk to the tor, the dress for our wedding had arrived. That seemed very auspicious. As I lifted it in delight from the box, beautiful silk covered in chrysanthemums emerged from the delicious tissue-paper wrapping. It fit! What a treat, to see my poor old body clothed in something so feminine and glamorous.

> Stringing beans in the late-autumn garden. The last crop. We had given up hope for them this year, but then came a late bumper harvest. We eat and share with surprised delight.

I became very aware at this time of how I always needed to do more. It was getting in the way of me relaxing, letting go, which I felt had been part of the cause of the illness. When I started doing Osho's meditations many years ago I had found them so helpful, letting go of physical stress before sitting in meditation. But in recent times I had done them less and less, always feeling there were more pressing things to attend to. And now it was difficult to do some of the more physically demanding ones, or even to sit still and meditate as my mind was so frantic. I knew I had to rediscover that peaceful, accepting space that I had experienced through meditation. I remembered times of sitting in front of Osho, meditating in Buddha Hall in the ashram, the deep peace and quiet joy. I wondered if that would ever be possible again. I longed to let go, to just be.

In the street one day we meet a Tibetan Buddhist monk. We get chatting, and I am in awe of his calm and presence. When he says to me 'You have a lot of strength in your gentle nature' I am very moved. I have never before thought of myself as a strong person. Perhaps I am finding some untapped parts of myself as I face this terrific fear. And perhaps facing that fear is part of my healing, my coming fully into my own being.

A healing session with Helen. I felt blissful. And as though I was expanding, really big, and glowing. Then I knew I was about to have one of those horrible hot, sweaty chemo moments, when a switch in my solar plexus seems to be suddenly turned on. I get a sense of dread when that happens, feel very vulnerable and soon afterwards the hotness comes. This time I just stayed with it, rather than throwing off layers of clothes, and actually it wasn't as bad as I feared. It quite soon passed. So maybe there's a lesson there, about witnessing, letting things pass through.

It's our wedding day. I have been worried that I'll be weepy all day, but there is too much happiness for that. Because I am weak from the treatment we have decided to just have a very small ceremony and lunch party, and to have a bigger celebration in summer.

Liz strews rose petals on the path in front of us as we leave the house. Jo and Fran join us at the registry where we giggle and shed a few tears. The ceremony is very moving. I give thanks for Chetan, for so much he has given to me in this life. We celebrate that, in the funny little registry office full of filing cabinets, flowers and office chairs.

Our guests participate in the ceremony by first reading out some words of Osho:

Love is the centre of life. Love is the very purpose, the destiny of life.

Then a beautiful poem from Christina Rossetti:

My heart is like a singing bird
Whose nest is in a water'd shoot;
My heart is like an apple-tree
Whose boughs are bent with thick-set fruit;
My heart is like a rainbow shell
That paddles in a halcyon sea;
My heart is gladder than all these,
Because my love is come to me.
Raise me a dais of silk and down;
Hang it with vair and purple dyes;
Carve it in doves and pomegranates,
And peacocks with a hundred eyes;
Work it in gold and silver grapes,
In leaves and silver fleurs-de-lys;
Because the birthday of my life
Is come, my love is come to me.

And that's exactly what I felt I was celebrating. That my love had come to me, my beloved Chetan. We had been friends for many years, since our mid-20s, and somehow he was always there at times of difficulty for me – and others too! It was Chetan who had introduced me to Osho. One day, after many years of friendship, my feelings for him changed and deepened. I'd suddenly seen how gorgeous he was too. Now, even though things could be scratchy and difficult between us at times, because we were in such unknown territory, the illness was showing me that love even more.

And from Rumi, a verse that's probably about god really, but love is love:

The minute I heard my first love story,
I started looking for you,
Not knowing how blind that was.
Lovers don't finally meet somewhere,

They are in each other all along.

Then to lunch at a gorgeous country hotel, where we find that Nigel has ordered champagne for us. What a really lovely thing to do. At the end of the fabulous lunch a wedding cake from Liz is brought in, to our surprise and delight. On the top of it little model figures of bride and groom make us laugh. Here we are, in our 50s, playing at being newly-weds and having the most joyful time!

Today is the start of a new part of my life. I let go of all I no longer need, and choose to live in joy and love.

There are so many cards from friends, filled with their love. I am full of good food, of happiness and laughter, shared friendship, and above all of love.

Next day I sit in bed and see my wedding bouquet on the windowsill, my lovely dress hanging up, a beautiful heart-shaped wreath studded with camellias from Ali hanging on the wall. I feel the preciousness of being there with Chetan, and give thanks to the divine for this great love in my life. I do not take it for granted, I know the difficulties and pain of relationships too, and how blessed I am now.

I don't stay in bed long. We're off to Cornwall in the caravan for our honeymoon! It might be only the end of March, but it's time to celebrate our marriage and getting through the long winter of chemo.

Two weeks in our little caravan, overlooking the stunning St Ives Bay. It was Chetan's birthday the day after we arrived, the sun shone and the sea was every shade of deep blue and aquamarine. We sat on the harbour front, soaking up the early April sun, and ate in a lovely café by the beach. Such delights after the difficult months. After our meal we walked on the beach. It was painful to see young families playing together, and knowing that I could barely walk, let alone run around like them. I felt the loss of that physical vigour I had once just taken for granted. But other than that, and the soreness in my feet and hands, I felt quite good physically.

Last night I dreamt about a seductive, attractive man trying to take me away from Chetan. I thought maybe that was about death. Sad.

It must have been very difficult at times for Chetan. I'd insisted on bringing the juicer with us, so that I could continue having fresh veg juice twice a day. Imagine doing all the veg preparation and cleaning the juicer in a small caravan! And he must have been very worried at times. When we visited the Tate gallery in St Ives I kept collapsing in a tearful heap, feeling so weak. In the second week I just had to rest a lot. Chetan told me later he thought perhaps I was dying.

But I wasn't. At least, no more so than that every day, every breath, takes us closer to death. I was starting to let that in.

We visited Gwynver Beach, the place where I had first started to sense that something was wrong. It was a strange, magical day. On the way along the spectacular coast road from St Ives to the foot of Cornwall we drove in and out of brilliant sunlight one moment and dense fog the next. The beach was shrouded in mist, but it was still wonderful, one of my favourite places in the world, and somewhere I'd often 'travelled' to in visualisations. I had wondered if it might be painful to return, but sitting on spray-soaked rocks with Chetan, taking photos of us huddled together in the mist, was joyful.

I made a little ritual design on the sand, a pattern of shells to bring light into the body and wash the disease away. I asked the ocean for this cleansing, and just as I was about to take a photo of my little icon a big wave came and washed it all away. The shells and water dispersed as though the pattern had never been.

I was delighted! It became a good visualisation for a while.

Being in Cornwall, a place I have known and loved all my life, brought it home to me. I was in a new place in my life. Fighting this was pointless. It was time to start accepting the situation. I realised this was different from resignation; it was about learning to live with this reality.

> *As the soft yield of water cleaves obstinate stone, so to yield with life solves the insoluble.*
>
> *– Lao-Tzu*

I dreamed intensely during those two weeks, perched in the van high above the Atlantic. One night I had a beautiful dream about Chetan, a joyful reunion after he had been abroad. Another night I dreamt of a strange animal that I was intensely interested in, only to realise it wasn't real at all, just a technological marvel I'd been wasting my time trying to feed. Was there a message there about having been preoccupied with things that weren't real or important at all?!

Our last day in St Ives. Very tearful for a while, not wanting to go into 'this may be the last time I come here', but it suddenly getting me. Gradually calmed down (thank you, Chet), and truly enjoyed sitting on the harbour beach, watching the kids play, the interplay of life and change, knowing that I too am part of it.

Chapter 10

I'm about to hear the results of the scan I had at the end of chemo. The results of all those months.

Another long, anxious wait in the gloomy waiting room. Then we're told that Dr Osborne isn't there, and we'll see her registrar instead. I've never met him before. It feels strange and disappointing to be seeing someone new at the end of this long stint. For me it's such an important meeting. What can he know about me?

I get the impression he has hastily looked at my notes before coming in. He seems to struggle to interpret the scan results, but apparently the liver tumours have reduced by about 50%. That's fantastic. More good news is that the CEA count in the blood has dropped hugely.

Yet somehow this young doctor makes it all sound very despairing. When I ask about the possibility of an operation he says, 'No one in the world would ever operate on your liver.' Does he need to put it so bluntly? What certainty he has, and what little hope he is giving me.

Then this young man tells me that there is nothing else that can be done until the cancer reactivates. 'Which will probably be at the end of summer,' he tells me.

I mention alternative treatments. He scoffs, saying that the iscador I am taking is 'just a poison' as it comes from mistletoe. It's not worth arguing with him, even though I'm tempted to say, 'So chemo isn't a poison then?' He tries to correct himself and pay some lip service to alternative treatments, maybe realising it's not great for a patient's morale. He tells me a story of a patient of his who has metastatic cancer and only comes in once a year for a check-up. But he doesn't know what this patient is doing right!

I come out of the meeting desperate just to leave the hospital. The news was much as I'd expected – both good and bad – but its delivery hadn't been helpful. I mustn't blame the messenger though, even though he could do with polishing up his technique in giving patients a bit of encouragement. Or any, really. I must find my own way.

On the way home I notice rowan trees on the moor. They are just coming into leaf. I picture them flowering in early summer, and the curdy blossoms later turning into scarlet berries. I wonder if I will see this happen. I feel so sad that I may not.

The rowan tree became a kind of symbol for me that summer. It was painful, watching the tree changing, and wondering. A bud opening up into a sturdy new leaf was both beautiful and dreadful.

I worked hard on building myself up.

I am calm and confident. My energy is focused and balanced. I am healing all the time.

I sought out anything that would buoy me up, give me hope and a sense that I had some part to play in this illness. The day after seeing this doctor the prayer from *Daily Word* was so apt:

> *I acknowledge the capacity for healing that is always present within every cell of my body. I cooperate with the creative power of God that brought me into being and is doing a healing work within me right now.*
>
> *Every day, in prayer, I bring into my consciousness a greater realisation of the power of God within me to heal and restore my mind and body. As I do, I participate in this healing, restorative activity, and I am healed in every way.*

It was time to start looking at the possibility of other treatments. The NHS's only offer was waiting for the cancer to reactivate, then hitting it with more chemo. But it seemed to me that this was exactly the time to be taking some sort of action. Couldn't I take advantage of the fact that the tumours and the cancer activity had reduced so much?

But how?

Outside my window a blackbird teeters on the end of a branch, gorging itself on ripe rowan berries.

I'd expected to feel much better once the chemo stopped, but it took quite a while. In fact I got more tired over the next few weeks, and my hands and feet burnt much more. Chemo goes on being active for two months or so after treatment has stopped, so I told myself that these symptoms were a good sign that it was still working. This was a time for recuperation, for letting the body heal and recover. I was more able to let myself take to my bed when the exhaustion overcame me.

Meditation is feeling a bit easier. It is the time for deepening that as much as I can, watching the fears and griefs, and coming back to the wonderful now whenever I can.

In my meditations I was so often wanting to get up and do something. Anything, rather than sitting there, going 'inside' where cancer was too. One time, crying while trying to meditate, I saw how much this wish to 'do' something was about running away from my feelings. In the sobs I saw a desire to die, to not have to deal with all the difficulties, the pain and fear of living.

This realisation that there is part of me that wants to die, that finds life such a struggle and so full of fear, was shocking. But I could feel it deep within me. Consciously I wanted – and want – to live, but there was a deep pull to die too. The idea of death could seem very attractive, the easiest place to be.

This was such an important insight. In past life work I could see that many lives of suffering had made me feel life was too unbearable, but how could I deal with that now? Even though that pull to death was there, on another level I had a really strong desire to live – to be in this body much longer, to love, to grow, to just be. Osho described what I was looking for:

> *Experiment with love in as many ways as possible and you will become richer every day. You will find new sources and new ways to love, new objects to love. And then ultimately a moment comes when one simply sits with no object of love, simply loving – just full of love, overflowing with love. And that is the state of enlightenment. One is fulfilled, utterly contented, one has arrived. The constant feeling that something is missing is, for the first time, no more there…*
>
> *My sannyasins are not to waste this opportunity. It has to be used to the full. We have to squeeze the juice of each and every moment to be the fullest!*

That was what I was seeking. To feel full of love and joy no matter what the circumstances; to learn to live consciously with this opportunity of being in a physical body. To squeeze the juice of life!

Though I now knew that part of me which wished for death, I also knew that I wanted to heal. I felt I was being told by great teachers that I could heal, I *can* heal.

At the end of April, about a month after I'd finished the chemo, I went to see Dr Rosy Daniel at her private practice in Bath. Having known her from when I worked at Bristol Cancer Help Centre, it was so good to see her again, and I felt such respect for the work she has done in looking at the many different approaches to cancer care.

Liz came with Chetan and me, a real supporter's meeting! And I did indeed feel supported. Rosy stressed the need to do something about the liver, to be proactive. She said that there were more options available for liver treatment these days than regional oncology often seemed to be aware of.

Surgery to the liver had, according to Rosy, really moved on recently. She said that some of the pioneers in this area were finding it difficult to get the message out there, that they could now do so much more. As well as surgery in which parts of the liver would be removed, she told us about ablation. This treatment in effect 'burns out' tumours using laser or radio frequency, with needles applied through the skin, rather than the abdomen being opened up. She saw this as a very possible and hopeful option, and gave us information about who to contact.

We came away from Rosy feeling that there was work to be done. Sitting in a little café together the spring sun shone in on us as we wondered if we dared hope a bit more. Was there really hope to be found in Rosy's suggestions? Would I be considered for such treatment, was it feasible, would the NHS back it? There were many questions to be asked, contacts to be pursued, judgements to be made. I was so thankful to have help with all this. And more was to arrive.

I planted sweet peas in the garden. So lovely to be out there, and I heard and even *saw* the cuckoo for the first time this spring. These last few days since seeing Rosy have been intense and challenging, realising we can and must now start investigating other options. But I think I'm coming back up again.

My energy was improving. A bit less exhaustion as I moved further away from the chemo.

I started being part of an art group at the Force cancer support centre in Exeter. I was now a participant, not the one running it. I knew this might be painful, but really wanted to have the chance to paint and draw with that kind of support. It was more difficult than I'd expected, feeling the loss of my previous work, which had been such a big and important part of my life. I was very sad. But doing the artwork was good. Now it was *my* time for painting, drawing, allowing myself to unfold through art.

One of my paintings was titled *In a different world now.*

Chapter 11

I was in new territory. Yet again. Rosy had spelled out the importance of getting treatment for the liver as soon as possible. But how would I judge what was the best thing? Would I be able to get any such treatment within the NHS, and what might the implications be if not? I didn't know if I could possibly manage to pay for private treatment. Also, at that time there was a very public discussion going on about patients being excluded from NHS treatment altogether if they went for any private 'top-up' care. This was a scary thought. Would I be launched into a world of no NHS support if I did opt for some private treatment? Whatever the shortcomings of the NHS, it at least seemed to offer a cradling of support.

The first thing, though, was to follow up Rosy's suggestions and see what might be available. I was still struggling with my energy though, which made investigating things so difficult.

I seem to be getting weaker, able to do less. I had thought that after the chemo I would gradually pick up, get stronger, but it doesn't seem to be like that now, and I don't know if it's temporary or permanent. I daren't think in terms of healing, of recovery, in case I'm actually going into the dying process. Oh God, how can I say that? I *want* to get better, I need to find faith and hope. Right now I don't feel that, though I know I'm surrounded by love.

And so the major part of investigating what treatments were available fell to Chetan.

The possibility of an operation on the liver through the NHS drew a blank.

So ablation looked like the only possibility. Unfortunately Dr Osborne said this was not possible at Exeter, even though there was a radiotherapy department there, or anywhere else in the NHS. She thought that the cancer would soon reactivate, and that as it was in the lymph a procedure to the liver was pointless.

I couldn't accept this. Rosy had given us a couple of leads and we decided to pursue them. One was Dr Alice Gillams, at University College Hospital, London. The other was Professor Vogl at Frankfurt University Hospital, Germany. We would approach them both. As non-medics this was such difficult territory – knowing where to go, what to say and above all to whom. It involved asking our GP for a referral, and swimming around in a sea of not-knowing.

Today I drew one of my Angel Cards that friends gave us on our wedding. It told me to release and surrender, to let the angels help, support and guide.

The message was spot on, but surrendering to what might happen was so difficult. Every day there would be new emails batted about, new avenues to pursue. Perhaps a request to another consultant, or seeking information and support from other medics, but all stemming from our own efforts.

We learned that Professor Vogl's treatment was to give chemotherapy direct into the liver via an artery. Known as chemoembolisation, this could shrink the tumours in the liver, hopefully with little debilitating effect on the rest of the body. Once the tumours had been reduced they would then be given laser ablation, to 'deaden' or calcify them.

I'd already been turned down for so many things, I didn't dare hope that I would be accepted for this treatment. And would it be the right thing to go for anyway?

Professor Vogl's staff at Frankfurt University Hospital were very efficient and helpful when we contacted them. They told me, to my astonishment, that the Professor himself would phone me that day. I waited on tenterhooks. Such a lot hung on this. He phoned.

Yes. Professor Vogl thought that he could do chemoembolisation, followed by ablation, on my liver.

At first I didn't feel elated. I had so desperately tried not to be too optimistic, to stay calm and centred, that I had almost cut myself off from the possible outcome in case it wasn't good. It wasn't really until the next day that it hit me. Yes, I *was* being offered this treatment. I felt I had been given divine guidance and support – and quite a bit of the human kind too.

A bit weak and tearful this morning, but sitting here in the garden I am so aware of my many blessings. A beautiful spring day, buds bursting open, the azaleas showing reds and purples, blossom on the cherry trees. News of an awful disaster in Burma brings it home even more. How blessed and cared for I am in this moment. I send my prayers to those people. Perhaps I can have more hope for the future. I pray that they can too.

A few days later I have an appointment with Dr Osborne. She again states that the cancer is likely to reactivate quite soon. Of course I rail against that, not wanting to hear what I know is likely, but needing to maintain my own hope and determination, to have faith in all I am doing too.

I need to talk with her about Professor Vogl's type of treatment. I hadn't expected a rather scathing dismissal of the idea. It is not provided in this country, she says, as it's unproven.

'Professor Vogl is a maverick,' she says.

When I say that I am thinking very seriously of having the treatment in Germany she is astonished. She makes it clear that the NHS would not even consider supporting me. She thinks that I should have more systemic chemo when the time comes, and if I'm still interested in the ablation option, to go for that then.

I reel out of the appointment, feeling that a rug has been pulled out from under me. Everything is suddenly up for question. She has told us there is no way the NHS would approve the treatment – that is, pay for it – and that she herself disapproves of it. We're on our own, both financially and in decision-making. Not to mention the possibility of being denied further NHS treatment if I go to Germany. Will I dare to jump out of the NHS cradle? Is she right, is Professor Vogl just a maverick? Is being a maverick a good or a bad thing? She was no more hopeful about the London option, just thought her own treatment was the right way, and that it was foolish to consider anything else.

I picture myself another few months down the line, feeling even worse after more systemic chemo. How would I possibly be able to deal with this German option then? I sense that if I'm going to have it, the time is now.

I felt like a statistic. That my possibilities of living or dying were being judged against statistics of expected outcomes. Which of course they were. But where was the possibility of things being anything other than predictable, of me as an individual?

I am not a statistic and am doing all sorts of things that may help. I do have to acknowledge the possibility of death, to live with both living and dying. I ask for guidance on what is best. So how to live today? Be joyful and grateful for this lovely day. Be thankful that I have another opportunity to grow in consciousness and awareness, to love and be loved, to feel myself with roots into the earth and wings in the divine.

But we were actually far from alone. To my great relief my cousin Martin was again on hand to help guide us through this medical morass. He helped us through making decisions about treatment. I was incredibly fortunate to have this support. Martin read through Professor Vogl's research reports, and his response was positive. Vogl is internationally renowned, he pointed out, with impressive credentials, research and outcomes. Yes, he was pioneering, but producing impressive results and increasing patients' lifespans.

Vogl may be a maverick, I thought, but aren't mavericks just people who push things on, the risk-takers and pioneers? I felt I'd rather be in that territory than the conservative one.

> Wild Irish weather, wind and rain lashing an Atlantic headland. Bright Tibetan flags bend low in the gale. In the night moonlight across calmed waters.

I was still hoping, though, that Dr Gillams at University College Hospital might offer me treatment. It would at least be in the NHS, and in this country.

Waiting to hear from UCH was difficult. It was hard to make other plans. I sought help in all I could find:

> *Rest in natural great peace*
> *This exhausted mind*
> *Beaten helpless by karma and neurotic thought,*
> *Like the relentless fury of the pounding waves*
> *In the infinite ocean of samsara.*
> *– Nyoshul Khenpo*

I'm sure I didn't fully understand these words at the time, but they were reassuring and calming.

One morning I woke with great emotional pain in my heart. The intensity was almost physical, red-hot. I soon 'saw' a river of molten lava flowing from a volcano, and the pain turned to anger. Then the volcano erupted furiously, ejecting matter from deep within it. I allowed myself to travel into the volcano, knowing that I would not burn, but was supported by two angelic beings. Still crying and in pain, I came to a dark tunnel. There was light ahead, but it took an excruciating length of time to reach it.

Eventually I was there, in the light, and was laid upon the ground. A being of great light came to me, and to my delight some cats stroked gently against me. Other beings of light came too, and loved ones from this light who had passed over. I was still in some pain, but then felt as though a silver river was running out of me, carrying away all the pain of leaving life. In this river I saw a huge fish, which for a while got stuck. I knew the fish represented all my attachments, the 'stuff' it is so hard to let go of, good things as well as bad. It seemed that my attachments were so huge that the fish couldn't move around. When I asked for help, this great fish turned into many small ones which could then leave my body. Slowly calm came, I was wrapped in caring arms and being told I am never alone.

I felt that I was seeing what dying would be like. But that it was also about that moment, the letting go and trusting, going through pain whilst being open to love and peace. I felt very raw, weak and wobbly.

Then Liz phoned. We talked of clothes and shopping. Just what was needed!

Next morning I affirmed:

I choose to live in joy
I am happy, healthy and healed
I love myself
I love life.

I had also been on another past life workshop. In it I had 'seen' myself as a Roman soldier, a rather unconscious, violent man. After his death he came to feel the pain of what he had done in his life and to realise that he needed to be a 'soldier of the spirit'.

I found it very difficult to return from the altered state in which I experienced this, and realised I had to make a definite choice. Almost as though I was also deciding whether to live or die right now. My choice gradually became clearer – to live as fully as possible in this body, now. That however long I had to live, being in a body is so precious. I felt very determined and clear, as though I had taken on some of the Roman soldier's quality.

I felt clearer and lighter. As though I could accept both life and death.

> Treatment in London tomorrow. Will I survive? In the train I overhear talk of shopping trips, of films and theatre. We speed through bright, flooded countryside.

I returned to Penny Brohn Cancer Care (previously my old workplace of Bristol Cancer Help Centre) for a two-day course. How strange it was to be there not as a therapist but as the one with cancer, the one aching to be supported, shown how to heal, longing to be held together as I fell apart.

In the few years since I had left, the organisation had moved to wonderful new premises in a Georgian mansion. Being in a different location made it easier to accept going back; the place was not redolent with memories.

I arrived early, and went into the meditation room. I lay on my back on the floor, alone in this light-suffused place, and my body racked with sobs. The enormity of what had happened to me in the last nine months came crashing down on me. When, eventually, the crying subsided I stared up at the old rafters. The knots in the wood made the shape of a serene, Buddha-like face. I didn't care if it was just my imagination, it made me feel safe and protected. Understood.

Being at PBCC gently carried me into being the one with cancer, the one who would need supporting by these lovely old friends of mine running the course. But I was still part of them too – I even found bits of my old writing in the art room. Two parts of my life – before and after cancer, which had felt like two pieces of severed cloth – were being sewn back together again. I was in a different world now, but I could feel love from my 'old world', showing me I was still valued for who I had always been, and continued to be.

I had thought that being with other people with cancer might be difficult. It was the opposite:

I'm so inspired by the other participants - the courage, how they've dealt with it. Both acceptance and fighting spirit. No, that's not quite right - more like determination to be with the present, to live as fully as possible. And that means different things for each of them, which is maybe another lesson too, about becoming more oneself.

There was M. who had survived ovarian cancer years longer than expected and whose husband brought her champagne in the bath. C., who had spent weeks in isolation following a bone marrow transplant and had set up an exhibition in his hospital room. T., who had just heard that cancer had spread to her kidneys and who faced an imminent prospect of leaving her children motherless. K., who still wore a bandana over her bald head but expected to return to work, and to what she saw as a new way of living, very soon.

Each of us had some extraordinary combination of fragility and fortitude.

I heard the sad news of the death from Parkinson's of one of the founders of BCHC, and of how in the last weeks he was barely able to communicate, but had continually recited the prayers he knew so well from having been a vicar. I was glad that he had had that solace. It also made me wonder what resources I myself had for dealing with imminent death. How would I cope? I knew I didn't have anything so deeply part of me. Other than Osho – but how could I access my connection with him when I was dying?

A few days later I hear that Dr Gillams has turned me down. She is kind and helpful, but says that because of the lymph involvement and the size of the tumours it is not possible to give radio frequency ablation. I could contact her again in a year's time, she says. Does she really think I'll still be here then? Can she possibly imagine that our paths will cross again?

So I am left with either waiting for summer to pass and the likelihood of more systemic chemo, or treatment in Germany.

Struggling to not sink into depression. Aware on waking of a great weight, feeling of hopelessness, the torture of having to decide about the German treatment.

Went down to feed the cats. Put on washing, stood outside and breathed in the lovely soft, fresh air. Brought the hazy sun into me, and felt the earth beneath me. Felt stronger.

All this decision-making has so dominated the last week or so. I need to get back to other things - to living in this beautiful summer, walking, seeing friends, but in a way that doesn't put more demands on Chetan. All those things are important too.

Chapter 12

The Bristol Channel lies far below. The two Severn bridges glint in the sunlight, and with a bit of wishful thinking I may even see my mother's house. We're on our way to Germany, for me to start treatment at Frankfurt University Hospital.

> Two magpies perch high in an autumnal tree. One for sorrow, two for joy. I am still here.

After months of being so much at home, air travel is a delight. Even the airport is exciting, and Chetan and I treat ourselves to a big breakfast as we wait for the plane at Bristol.

As the plane rises high, we look down on pillowy sunlit clouds. It's as though all those visualisations of light I've done while lying in bed are manifesting themselves. Coming in over Frankfurt I wonder about the lives of the people in the many tiny houses below us. How different or similar they may be to mine. I feel connected to this great world again, back in the play of life.

It had been a big decision. In choosing to come to Germany for treatment I was turning my back, at least for the moment, on what the NHS had to offer. I cannot claim much credit for all the work and research that went into making the decision. My brain still went into meltdown as soon as I sat at the computer or attempted reading anything vaguely technical. Chetan had read through articles by Professor Vogl about his work, and Martin had been very much part of the research and decision-making process. I took in as much of the technical information as I could. Professor Vogl's work certainly indicated better prognosis for someone in my situation, and to my very unscientific mind it made sense to apply chemotherapy direct to the liver, followed by laser treatment.

In the end, though, I had to go on what my heart and body felt, just as much as on what my mind could comprehend. I just knew it was the right thing for me. If I was taking a step away from the NHS, I was also seizing hold of my own process.

> The river has burst its banks, unable to contain a whole November's rain. Cold, damp air strikes my face as I walk beside it. I run a few paces, the first since summer.

It also meant a big leap of faith financially. We hoped we could persuade the NHS to pay, but meanwhile had to find substantial sums of money. I could expect to have between two and six chemoembolisations, costing about £3,000 each, followed by one or two laser ablations each costing twice that.

We didn't have anything like that kind of money, but we could manage the first payment.

Do I dare hope? A little bit of me urges caution - what if I get there and they change their mind?

If Rosy's right, maybe one day an op on the colon might even be possible.

The journey since the diagnosis has been such a huge one that I dare not hope too much - though having that sense of hope is wonderful too! A strong voice in me is saying to stay centred, keep doing my inner work, remember all I've been learning. Yes - to also enjoy life, being alive, the delights of life too.

I had become more aware of the preciousness of small things – a blue sky, a little teddy bear with angel wings given to me by my nephew Joe, a woodpigeon flying in a blue sky, the sound of Chetan in the kitchen. So many things to be grateful for, if I only looked.

Stay centred. Choose to live in joy. Stay in your own power, work with your inner healing.

I had come to know – or at least be open to the possibility – that I do have spirit guardians. A session with the clairvoyant Dorothy Chitty had shown me that one of my guardians was a 19th century German doctor, very interested still in all things medical. I had sometimes felt him during a healing session, and as we approached Frankfurt Hospital I had a strong sense of him almost rubbing his hands in eager anticipation.

Dorothy had also said to me, 'You can get through this'. I could only hold out my hands in hope, and pray that she was right.

Frankfurt Hospital is elegant plate glass, gleaming marble and steel, very different from the hospitals I have been in so far. It sits on the edge of the wide river Main, and we have walked along the riverbank to get there early in the morning. I have not slept well, fearful that I'll be told something like the cancer has spread too far, it's no longer treatable. Walking up from the river towards the imposing entrance, I can see that just inside is a huge suspended sculpture which reminds me of angels' wings. I ask that all beings who are with me will help me heal, and I sense my German doctor guardian looking round with incredulous eagerness.

Professor Vogl is tall, brisk, kindly, matter of fact. And very busy. We learn later that he often gets to the hospital at 4am, and he is clearly extremely dedicated to his work. I like him, though he's a little scary too. He explains what he hopes to achieve with the treatment, and says that the chemoembolisation will treat not only the liver, but will affect the lymph too, and that perhaps eventually the colon could be operated on. I scarcely dare to believe it, to hope.

A nurse takes me into a tiny cubicle to change into a hospital gown before the procedure. I have to wait a while, and try to stay focused, to relax my breathing, to just be with being alone, feeling vulnerable in this closet. A nurse comes to check through my details. He is Egyptian, and perhaps feels some connection for someone who is also away from their homeland. Whatever the reason, after doing the medical bits he talks to me about the importance of having hope, of seeing myself getting well. I still feel grateful to him.

There are scans and blood tests, then I lie on what looks like an operating table. A canula is put into my vein, through which dye will be injected so that a scanning device can allow Professor Vogl to insert a tube through the artery, up into the liver where chemo drugs will be deposited and plugged in place.

Professor Vogl comes into the room once I'm prepared. He talks kindly to me, whilst very clearly focusing on what he is doing. A nick in my groin is slightly painful, then the tube is inserted. It's uncomfortable, but nothing too bad. I've been given a sedative, and become quite groggy. I'm aware that Professor Vogl is watching the tube's journey, and my liver, on monitors which I can also see. But I don't want to watch. I just try to stay calm, to feel that healing is coming to me.

I'm wheeled out into the recovery room, groggy and slightly nauseous. In and out of sleep, I'm aware of Chetan coming in to see me. How lovely. I'm there a few hours, gradually drinking, eating some dry biscuits, coming to and feeling very cared for by the nurses.

Just a few hours after this procedure we're heading back to the hotel. I'm feeling very delicate, but happy. I stay in bed while Chetan ventures into Frankfurt to eat. How wonderfully he looks after me, bringing me just a little something to tempt my appetite.

> Dazzling winter sunshine through clifftop-high spray from wild Cornish waves. It is my third Christmas since finding I am ill. The beach is alive with people, dogs, horses and us.

I have to return to the hospital next morning for a scan. As we walk along the riverbank (yes, I actually feel well enough to walk the half-mile) we see a pair of geese with a family of tiny goslings. I've never seen geese quite like them, and the little group lifts my spirits. Professor Vogl says I will need to return for the next treatment in a month. He also says that I will need to take an oral chemo drug – it's the more low-level one I'd taken while on chemo before. He tells me I will need to obtain this from my UK consultant.

Back home. I walk up the garden path, giving thanks for my safe return, and am greeted by the two cats. I feel pretty good.

I dreamt I was staying in a hotel room. Suddenly noticed that two people, a rather shabby man and woman, had moved into the room along with lots of baggage. I was furious, asked them how they dared without even asking. I pushed them firmly out of the door - they seemed a bit bewildered, couldn't understand what the problem was. Then I started chucking out all their baggage - there was lots, I kept finding more. Then they seemed to accept being chucked out. I wasn't sure if a couple of things belonged to them or the room, but they seemed like treasures so I kept them in the room.

I wonder if this was about cancer invading me. I am so outraged that it has. And now I *am* throwing it out - yes, *it can go*. Maybe the 'treasures' were to do with the learning that has happened through it - they were old-fashioned instruments for gaining knowledge and wisdom.

I also dreamt of a young baby and wanted to care for and protect this beautiful, precious little thing. Is this about loving that part of myself, the innocent, vulnerable me?

Chapter 13

One of the many people who had given me a lot of support since my diagnosis was Dr Annie Paxton. She had been a consultant haematologist, and after retirement became very interested in alternative methods of healing. I met her when she came to work at Bristol Cancer Help Centre and we had stayed in touch afterwards. When I was diagnosed she gave me such sensible advice – to rest lots, eat what I fancied, take some vitamins and worry about all the rest after chemo. Coming from someone who had been a top-notch consultant and was now very interested in contacting cosmic sources for healing assistance, I loved this down-to-earth advice. It was like being given permission to just rest, relax, take care of myself.

One day a letter arrived from Annie. She had received a 'channelled' message from the astral beings who, she said, were teaching her about healing. The message was about painting:

This soul needs to really look into her fear. Sometimes it weighs heavy and is a barrier to her well-being. Her disease is resting at the moment, but is only resting. She is at the moment keeping it at bay. What she sees as perhaps inevitable does not have to be if she can deal with this fear. It is when she piles fear upon fear that we have difficulty helping her.

She can paint it out. She has the help at her own fingertips. There is a deep-rooted anger there that she will find she has not identified yet, that has been with her for most of her life, that she has been suppressing and that is the root of her illness.

The chemicals will affect the function of the liver, and she will feel very poorly at some stage and then the fear will surface. To distract yourself from fear is not dealing with it. In dealing with fear all humans work differently. This soul has the ability at her fingertips that she could use, to paint and find the anger at the base of it. She must not allow herself to lead the painting, she must allow the painting to lead her.

So it seemed it was now time to use my art much more fully for myself. I had done some artwork in the last few months, but it had been mainly rather lacking in energy; it didn't have real drive and let-go behind it.

Annie's letter seemed to throw a switch in me. I immediately went upstairs, found some paints, grabbed some bits of old card, and started painting furiously. And fury is exactly what it was.

A floodgate had been opened. I would only have to pick up a paintbrush to start crying, screaming, shouting. I painted on thick paper to start with – sheet after sheet. Mostly just furious scrubbing, scratching, flicking paint, layer upon layer. Usually words would come to me as I painted, expressing my anger and grief. Sometimes these got incorporated into the work, otherwise I wrote them on the back. Some images would end up with many such 'titles'.

I would often wake in the morning full of emotion, or memories of a bad dream. Chetan would encourage me to go and paint, there and then. I would fling on a scruffy old dressing gown which became increasingly encrusted in paint, filled my water pot, and emerged an hour or so later after often quite harrowing work. Chetan would be there in the kitchen; he must have heard all the screams and shouts, but quietly say 'well done', hug me and give me my porridge.

> Powdery snow lies thick on iron-hard ground. A distant hill is pink-bright against dark metallic sky. I leave my tracks in the fresh fall, privileged to be the first.

I discovered my late father's paint box, complete with his name inside it. Perhaps he was encouraging me in this. I've always loved art materials, like a kid in a sweet shop, so filling the paint box with some new paints was a real treat.

Within the first month or so of this outpouring I had made about thirty paintings on paper. I switched to painting on some boards which had been in a cupboard with half-finished pictures on them for years. I painted over the old images, not caring about losing something that had seemed important aesthetically. This was *my* time now. I didn't care what they looked like, it was all about the process. There was freedom in this, even within the rage and sorrow that poured out.

I played loud music. I yelled. I howled. I threw paint around with force and abandon. I was very lucky to live with someone who gave me the space for this, didn't seek to come and comfort me, but trusted in what I was doing. But knowing that Chetan was there was part of it too. He soothed the rawness telling me I was doing wonderful work, and I would be astonished by his endurance and understanding of what must have seemed quite crazy.

In time I moved on to painting on canvas too. I'd always felt very self-conscious about that, thinking it had to be something really good if it was on a canvas. Now it was my playpen, to leap around in as I wished.

Soon after my first treatment in Germany I had an appointment with Dr Osborne. Professor Vogl had told me that I would need to take some oral chemo to support the chemoembolisation, and that I should get it from my UK consultant.

Dr Osborne has two support nurses with her, as though she needs protection or witnesses. It doesn't feel nice. She is astonished that I have gone ahead with the treatment despite her view. She probably can't support me with chemo, she says, and is clearly angered by Professor Vogl's request. I can understand she would wish this to come direct from him, but am taken aback by several scathing backhanded comments about the treatment. She thinks I have done the wrong thing.

When I said that Professor Vogl had suggested a colon operation might be an option eventually, she said, 'Oh yes, we've always seen that as an option.' But that's a *lie*. She's only ever talked about a stent or a bypass stoma, not *removal* of the cancer. How dare she. I am exploding with anger.

I leave the hospital, incandescent with rage. I feel totally undermined. I can understand that she has a different opinion but *I* am the patient, the one with a life-threatening condition. Is it too much to expect support, for my decisions to be honoured, to be compassionate about my choices? Professional opinion is of course important, but it is my – the patient's – right to choose, and to hope for support in this. But I know that support is not really there. Mother Oncologist has chucked me out of the NHS nest because I won't 'be good'. What childhood stuff has this unearthed!

Thank goodness I could let all this out through painting. After the appointment I got on the train to go to Liz's for a few days, thankful I'd packed my paints.

Even in the midst of my rage I knew there was a lesson here for me. If I'd been cast into outer darkness by Dr Osborne, it was because I'd rebelled, I'd made my own choice. Despite the doubts she had sown, I still felt it was the right option for me. I was coming to realise that even if I 'rebelled' there are many sources of love and support that are always unconditionally there.

I asked for help and 'saw' a hot air balloon taking away these difficult feelings. It moved so slowly, such a weight. Eventually, out over the sea, it dropped to the depths of the ocean where it would be taken care of harmlessly.

And now to bring in the light, the love, that's my work.

Annie, through her guides, soon confirmed that my choice of the German treatment was the right one. Everyone has their own agenda, she was told in relation to Dr Osborne. And the message was also that chemoembolisation will be the way ahead for such treatment in the future.

My stay at Liz's was wonderful. Sharing with her, feeling so supported and loved, enjoying being with her, Tom, Joe and Paul. Joe even let me have a go on his mini-motorbike. Wobbling around the lawn on it, I was reminded of the sense of freedom I'd had as a teenager when I got a moped. There was still life in the old girl after all!

Chapter 14

A day I thought I might never celebrate again – my birthday. I'm 56, and resolve that this will be the best year of my life, so far. We celebrate in Lyme Regis, where a torrential thunderstorm sends waves crashing over the seafront.

What I want for my birthday is to *live without fear*. As that's a negative, what's the positive? *Live in love. Live in trust.*

When the weather clears we lie in sheltered dunes, a soft, sandy hollow with long grasses, listening to the sea. Chetan puts his hand over my heart, and fear and sadness melt as I sink into the warm sand, the strong wind, the smell of the sea, the sound of the gulls.

I was having occasional glimmers of facing death with less fear. At times! There was still a lot of grief about leaving life, and fear about the dying process, but sometimes a glimpse of equanimity. And, increasingly, knowing that I am loved which seemed to open a door to accepting myself, my life, and one day my death.

> A huge flock of geese wheels in ragged v-formation over snow-covered fields. Where can they find food in this harsh winter? I am warm and well-fed. I have travelled safely across the moor. On my way for another scan.

The second trip to Germany arrived and this time Liz came with me. Plenty of anxiety again – was the treatment doing any good, and if not would Professor Vogl turn me away… But there was great fun and joy in being with Liz too, almost as though we were on holiday, at least on the way out. The evening before the procedure we strolled along the river in summer sunshine, eating ice cream. The geese were still there – all their little ones had survived a month on this great river, and I took it to be a good omen.

Another treat was staying in a hotel which overlooked the River Main, watching the huge barges, and the city lights at night. It was just a business hotel, but we soon got to know which room to ask for to get this penthouse view.

As I emerged groggily from the procedure, Professor Vogl told me that the first session had reduced the liver tumours by ten to fifteen per cent. Great joy. My only real difficulty had been feeling very nauseous when the contrast dye for the scan was injected into my veins. An allergic reaction to the dye would make it difficult for the tube into the liver to be placed. I resolved to work on this reaction, to find ways of reassuring my body so that it didn't go into shock.

The return journey was difficult – or could have been if Liz hadn't been so together. A problem with Lufthansa meant we might not be able to fly that day at all, but with Liz's persistence they came up with a flight that was leaving imminently, and would just mean we had to change at Brussels. But there were only minutes to get this new flight. Frankfurt Airport is huge, and the terminal was half a mile away! Liz corralled a passenger buggy to whizz us down to the terminal. Strange, being now the 'disabled' person you see being whisked through security and departure. But wonderful – we made the flight.

It was all pretty exhausting, after the treatment and compounded by the change at Brussels Airport, surreally packed with some lovely original artwork and what looked like the world's entire collection of Belgian chocolate. It was a relief to get back to Bristol, but we hadn't been able to contact Chetan to tell him how and when we would arrive so that he could collect us. It turned out he had had a problem with his mobile. By some miracle he was driving right past the exit as we came out – another little gift of synchronicity. I said goodbye to dear Liz with great gratitude.

On the way home Chetan and I stayed for a few days with Fran and Jonathan. We sat in a sunny July garden, resting, enjoying friendship. Fran gave us both a reflexology session as we reclined in the sun, which really helped the discomfort in my abdomen. They took us to a 'performance' of Tibetan Buddhist prayer and chanting. Perhaps a seed was planted then. The Tibetan Buddhist monks affected me deeply, with their commitment to their way of living. As we returned home, from Germany, from being with our dear friends, from seeing the Buddhist monks, I had a sense of entering into a new phase of my healing.

> *God's spirit abides and thrives within me, regardless of what is happening in my life. In sweet moments of meditation, I nurture a growing awareness of God's love for me and within me, and healing is the natural result. God's love is within every cell of my body.*
> *– Daily Word*

Perhaps I should add that by 'God' I simply mean the divine, the source of all from which this extraordinary universe emanates. For me God is a useful tag sometimes, allowing access to many wisdom teachings but not limiting from where I may wish to learn.

A special occasion was approaching. We had decided to celebrate our wedding with our family and friends when I was a bit recovered from chemo, and the celebration was soon. We hoped to have a picnic by the river for about sixty people, but that would depend on the weather. Sun on Dartmoor is not guaranteed, so the village hall was the backup.

First, though, another trip to Dr Osborne to see if she would continue to support me while I was having treatment in Germany, or if I should ask for a referral to another consultant. I felt that when I'd last seen her I'd been so taken aback by her response that I hadn't found the words to say what I thought. So

I worked hard on what I wanted to say – that I wanted her to support my decision even if she didn't agree with it, that it was my choice, and I didn't want any implications that I'd brought it on myself if I ran into difficulties. I managed to say this clearly and hopefully without rancour as I felt very grateful for what she had done for me previously. Dr Osborne said she was happy to monitor me, and to take me 'back on board' after I'd finished the Germany treatment, but again said she could not give me the additional chemo tablets Vogl said I needed.

I sensed she was still quite angry with my decision, and I felt it was time to seek out another consultant. I feel great gratitude to her for all she did for me in those first months – she was kind, rooting for me, but it was time to move on. She offered to make a referral to another consultant.

It felt scary, but I trusted that it was for the best and that I was going into a new phase of healing.

I feel good that I was able to be forthright, proud and dignified. I would truly love to find an oncologist who will support me through their attitude - including knowing rather more about *me*, who I am and what will truly help my healing, as well as being open and supportive of my choices now or in the future.

I can still feel it lingering a bit, so now I need to let it go, trust that the perfect treatment and healing are already in place. Thank you for the healing.

Yet again I was so glad to be able to hurl paint at canvas.

When we'd arranged our marriage celebration I hadn't realised the date was exactly a year to the day since my diagnosis. What a strange and wonderful coincidence.

For days before the celebration there was torrential rain. The ground was sodden, the river almost overflowing. We still held out a slight hope of a bright day, and a sunny picnic, but it had to be the village hall. When Paul, Joe, Tom and Chetan went to set up though, they discovered the hall was strewn with the previous night's cans, bottles, dirty plates and glasses. Those crazy partygoers had planned on clearing up in the morning. But it soon looked lovely thanks to our dynamic cleaning crew. Liz had brought armfuls of flowers which decorated the trestle tables. Everyone brought wonderful food to share; we felt wrapped in love. I felt overwhelmed by everyone coming to be with us, and all they did. Embarrassed at times, to be the centre with Chetan of so much attention, and feeling it was all a bit horribly impromptu – which it was – but realising the love that was there for us. A few days later I wrote:

The power of that day is still with me, it gave me such a sense of support, of being held. It's like in one of my pictures which I'd titled 'show me how to be like a little baby' - I think that's what it meant, to feel the love and strong, strong support that was just palpable on that day. And sometimes I really do need that. I love life, I love my wonderful friends and family. Of course I wobble at times, but I'm finding a greater calmness, and resolution.

And then the next day I was raging in my journal, that I couldn't find peace, and was almost hysterical with sorrow, grief and fear. That's how it went. Strength, frailty. Hope, despair. Joy, total grief.

Equanimity often felt like a remote aspiration. Even a trip with friends Shelagh and Ali to see the film of *Mamma Mia!* was like that. I loved the joy of it, and remembered many fantastic trips to Greece, but wondered if I would ever manage to go again. Shelagh and Ali seemed to just understand that, when I burst into tears on the way out, and hugged me close. I felt petty at being upset, rather than grateful for what had been, but it was just another step in realising I couldn't take anything for granted any more. Perhaps I'd go to Greece again one day, but perhaps not.

Inside an ancient cathedral the roof vaults high above me, holding histories of prayer, of tears, of reverence. I cry as I face more illness. Yet I am indeed held.

Financial matters loomed large. How were we going to pay for the treatments? And now there was the probable additional expense of paying for the extra chemo drug.

Yet again I can only think that divine help was with us. Slowly we managed. A legacy gradually came through, and I was able to access my various little bits of pension on the grounds of terminal illness. I know that Chetan had to present my 'terminal' status to the pension companies, and between him and the GP I was spared those excruciating conversations. Family members were very generous, as were some wonderful friends. But each time a treatment approached we would be scratching around for where the funding would come from.

Dr Osborne had said it was very unlikely that the NHS would pay for my treatment. It would require her backing for them to even consider it. Which of course would not be forthcoming.

Chetan wrote to the PCT to ask for funding, but was refused almost by return of post. He even went to see our MP, who was sympathetic but reiterated that our case was not likely to succeed without a consultant's backing.

Perhaps a new consultant would be more interested.

The only option for getting the chemo tabs was to buy them privately. Our local chemist was so dismayed at me having to pay for them that he sweetly gave a discount, but it was still a lot more money to find every month.

I dream about cancer cells. A voice is saying, 'We know who you are and we're closing in on you.' They were being rounded up, just like by a posse of goodies in a movie!

The third treatment in Germany went well. I didn't feel sick, as I had both times before; in fact I recovered from the treatment more quickly. Perhaps it was from telling my body it was safe, it didn't need to try to jump out of the way of what was being done to it, or perhaps it was the homeopathy I took. We walked along the river, the family of geese all still there, and up into the old town. It was fun getting to know our way around Frankfurt. My mother had come to stay here with a pen pal just before the war, and stayed lifelong friends with her, so there was a feeling of connection.

I had hoped that this might be my last chemoembolisation. It was going well, Professor Vogl told me, but I needed more.

Chapter 15

A little girl is crying for her mother, who does not come. After my fourth chemoembolisation in Germany I wake up in the recovery ward to the soul-wrenching sound. The ward is solely for people undergoing similar treatment to mine. What agonies has this child already gone through, what lies ahead of her in her life? In the bed opposite a beautiful young woman is being violently sick, though at least her family is with her.

What right did I – do I – have to complain about having cancer, dealing with treatment, facing death? I often felt that I really did have little reason to. I'd lived a relatively long, healthy and prosperous life compared with so many others.

But although I genuinely felt that way, it didn't always help with my own inner struggle. Perhaps our culture is so out of touch with death and dying that it makes facing our mortality very difficult.

The morning after the treatment in Germany I always had to return to the hospital for a scan and to see the Professor. Leaving the hotel I glimpsed myself in a mirror in the lift. In the confined space there was no escape from my image. I seemed to have aged overnight, my face puffed and red from steroids, drawn and tired.

Let out the pain and love will fill the space.
– Bernie Siegel

Although I had almost passed out after this treatment, once we were home I soon felt quite well, as I had before. It was a time of intense dreams, lots of them about anxiety and loss. One dream, featuring a lovely young man who wanted to seduce me, became an ongoing one in various different guises. In the dream I would be tempted to go off with this man, then suddenly realise that I was with Chetan, loved him and wanted to stay with him. The seductive young man was, I was sure, death. Perhaps death was indeed seductive and desirable at times, but actually I really wanted to be with Chetan still – I wanted to live.

This beautiful world
Shimmering in ecstasy

I dreamt about making a speech at my father's funeral, being worried I wouldn't be able to make my voice heard, but finding a way of doing so. Perhaps I was, through opting for this treatment, in some way finding my own voice.

> *However many times you fall, stand up. However many times you come close to despair, go on trusting. However many times your heart wants to close, keep it open.*
> *– Thuksey Rinpoche*

There were trips to the coast, enjoying a simple delight of sitting in a pub for lunch – and being able to eat it. A visit from a young friend, very pregnant with her second child, was a joy:

Sophie with her huge pregnant belly, so full of new life. Me being very aware of being in a very different place in my life, but accepting that and loving seeing them. And then a beautiful Beethoven prom on TV - how blessed we are to be able to hear such wonders. Dear Sophie... such mysteries, the great cycles of life, death, regeneration, destruction, rebirth.

A more difficult meeting was with Neera, a fellow sannyasin. I didn't know her well, but had heard her singing in the ashram and just loved her strong, soaring voice. She had recently moved to Devon, having been diagnosed with cervical cancer which had metastasised. We spoke on the phone, exchanging experiences, and would sometimes meet at a party or meditation. There was tenderness and empathy between us, but perhaps a wariness of getting too close. What if she dies before me, how will I cope? What can I offer without seeming to say I've got all the answers when our situations are very different? But also eagerness to hear the other's discoveries and ways of coping. Neera continued sharing her wonderful voice and music with us, and I would be deeply moved by what poured forth from her. It was full of life yet deep with stillness.

Walking by the river one day I found a rock beneath which I felt I'd like my ashes to be buried. Some time later I showed it, with difficulty for us both, to Chetan.

And at last some sunshine.

Being in bed is sometimes wonderful! It's evening, have come to bed early as I've been very tired. Through the window I see the bright half-moon in the twilight sky, on the radio Mozart, and candles and essential oils burning in the bedroom.

I go to see a new oncologist, Dr Francis Daniel (not to be confused with Dr Rosy Daniel) at Plymouth hospital. Going to a new hospital is good, there's less to trigger all the 'hospital stuff'; but after Frankfurt it seems so run-down, crowded and tatty. I notice that people going in for chemo have to take a ticket and wait for their number to be called, as though they're waiting at the supermarket deli counter. It seems so impersonal.

Dr Daniel is friendly and helpful, but in a difficult position. It is painful to go through my history again, having to acknowledge that my condition is so serious. Dr Daniel doesn't deride my decision about Germany, though is careful not to endorse it either. He's quite upfront, and I feel quite good about him. But when I broach the possibility of one day being able to have an operation on the colon, he holds out very little hope. Would I really want to spend a lot of time recovering from a major operation, he asks me. The implication is clear: I don't have much time, so why waste it like that? He also isn't able to prescribe the capecitabin, but offers to see me again when the treatment in Germany has finished. I tell him I don't want to know my prognosis, which he honours, but he clearly sees it as pretty limited.

Somehow I have to live with that, to accept that's their view, to know it's possible whilst also maintaining hope. It *is* possible I may live a long time yet, and of course I'm trying to manage that in all I do. But there's much more to it too. It's to do with the way I live every day - being the best I can, expanding my being, loving, being as alive as I can, having gratitude for all I have, doing nourishing, life-expanding things. Be joyful, be hopeful, be fully in life.

I was learning too to juggle the pull to death with the wish to live. I could see that at times I did want to die; it was all too much. 'What's the point?' summed it up painfully, even while another bit of me rejoiced in life. Accepting them both seemed the only way, although I was scared that acceptance of a wish to die would make it happen.

There was, though, plenty to balance out any wish to leave this life soon.

The printmaking workshop to which I had been going for years held an exhibition, as part of which other printmakers donated work to be sold in aid of my treatment. I was so moved by their offer – I didn't even know all of the artists who donated work. It made me feel part of another group of caring people, part of the world again. On the opening evening I went to the show, which was packed. Long rows of prints pegged up on washing lines, friends drinking punch, chatter and laughter in evening sun. I could hardly sleep that night for joy and gratitude.

When later a cheque came to me from the money raised, I was astonished by the amount. It was a huge contribution towards a treatment. And perhaps just as important was the overwhelming feeling of support from their kindness.

> Snow lingers round the field-edges, but shoots push up through sodden earth. I've just had bad news, yet I feel so happy in this moment. Gratitude for being here is a jewel I am glimpsing.

What, I wondered, should I be doing with this part of my life which would give me a sense of fulfilment and purpose. I asked for direction in a dream. That night I dreamt of being in a sunny art room, chatting with friends, with only a short time to the end of the lesson. I knew I was supposed to take art materials to the other side of a river I could see, but when I saw the river was flooded I was relieved that I didn't have to do it, that I could just stay chatting. But something didn't feel right, I hadn't fulfilled a 'duty' to take the art materials. When I looked again, the river wasn't flooded any longer, and I now felt relieved that I could take the art things across.

The dream was telling me that I needed to work much more fully with my art – to not make excuses, but to use it and do it, otherwise I would be unfulfilled. I had asked for guidance, I now needed to follow it, and it could inspire and teach me. I needed to cross that river!

After the fourth chemoembolisation Professor Vogl told me that the good news was that the right lobe of the liver was now quiescent, but that there was still activity in the left lobe. More chemoembolisation would be needed before the laser ablation was possible.

Before the next treatment, though, a treat was in store. A local cancer support charity, Lifeline Resources, offered us a weekend of respite. Its aim was to give people who had gone through treatment a time of nourishment for mind, body and soul and they certainly achieved it.

The weekend was held in Sharpham House, a stunning Georgian mansion overlooking the Dart Estuary. We were a group of about ten, all women apart from Chetan. There was fantastic food cooked specially for us, meditation, group work, time to just hang out and be. And all in this fantastic place, full of beauty and redolent with meditation and a commitment to ecology.

As I cautiously picked up a beautiful piece of modern pottery from a highly-polished mahogany table in a perfectly proportioned oval dining room, I felt that my life was being validated. I wasn't just a statistic who could be shunted along a dismal corridor leading only to imminent death; I was someone whose life had meaning and fullness, both in the past and now.

I take with me from this time feeling connected to life, a will to live. Knowing that I am part of a wonderful flow of life - the river, the yew tree, the house, the people, the beauty of the land and art, and that I *am* still connected to all that. The joy of being with others, the depth of sharing which makes me realise I'm not alone, I'm part of the flow of life.

I still feel grateful to the people who run this charity. It gave me back a feeling of worth, that my life was still valued. In the days following it there were still dreams about losing Chetan, such as not being able to phone him; but a little more joy in the present too. A beautiful early October morning in the garden, the sun still hot, a butterfly landing on the thyme flowers. Realising the simple pleasure of coming down in the morning, when I felt good enough, to feed the cats, put washing on, boil the kettle. Just being there. Light on the hill, mist in the valley, dewdrops on the wires and leaves, the start of another day.

What will you give
When death knocks at your door?
The fullness of my life –
The sweet wine of autumn days and summer nights,
My little hoard gleaned through the years,

And hours rich with living.
These will be my gift.
When death knocks at my door.
– Rabindranath Tagore

Chapter 16

Liz doesn't recognise me for a moment. I'm sitting in a wheelchair, and momentarily she sees Chetan but not me. When she looks down and does see me, I see the shock in her face. I guess I look pretty awful.

I'm being pushed through Heathrow Airport, on our way back from the fifth treatment in Germany. Feeling pretty rough, but I've made it back thanks to Chetan's help.

We had travelled from Heathrow this time so that before going we could attend a lecture in London on Jung by Roger Woolger. It was so exciting to be in London, full of life and activity – it still felt exciting to be out *anywhere*. I could hardly believe I was staying just round the corner from the British Museum. To our delight it was open in the evening, and we walked in awe around the new atrium and into the Egyptian sculpture gallery. Again that feeling of being still part of the richness of life. I looked in wonder at the huge lion-headed figures – what did these ancient people know of life and death that we may have lost?

Unfortunately this fifth treatment in Frankfurt affected me much more than usual. I was sick, with pain in the abdomen. The sickness went on for some days, needing medical intervention as I could keep nothing down and was getting dehydrated. We stayed at Liz's for a few days more than we had planned, until I was up to travelling.

It took ten days or so to recover, and to feel less weak. The soggy autumn seemed to reflect my own sense of sinking deep into mud and decay where only gruesome, rotting things dwelt. But there was also one night when, though still unwell, every time I woke up I felt as though my whole being was utterly peaceful, and that I was covered in a sparkling autumnal dew in golden light. I seemed to be pervaded by this beauty all night.

> Bantry Bay, a vast expanse of calm water beneath a clear spring sky. The sun rises over the mountain across the bay, first red then blazing yellow, diamonds dancing across the water. A half-moon still hangs in the sky. All is complete.

I needed to be starting on the capecitabin again, but couldn't face it. I dreamt of Sarah Palin as the wicked witch of the north, chasing me all over the place to take my chemo tabs.

I still wonder if this painful episode of physical illness was working on other levels too. Whilst in London I had also had a therapy session with Roger Woolger. In it I had seen generations of women on my mother's side who were furious about how they had been treated as women, sidelined, affected by wars, and frustrated by not being able to fulfil their potential. Perhaps this 'bile' had come down to me through generations of raging women, and was being released in this very unpleasant way. Certainly so much distress has been built into our culture that the wish to not be in the body is endemic, and I could see that for these women it resulted in bitterness and resentment.

But the session had also shown me life-affirming aspects of myself. I saw vibrant, lively figures who were keen to engage with me – through artwork. They were like alchemists, brewing up something potent that needed to be realised.

There was also a sense of contact with my father's father, who died before I was old enough to remember him. He was holding out an apple to me, clearly wanting to support me, and saying, '... when you die, whenever that is, it's really important that you know your life is as rich, full and matured as this apple is. Don't have regrets, it *is* ripened and rich.' He was laughing about his symbol, because he had called the house he built Little Orchard, so he was indicating what he had created, and that I too had created richness in my life.

Roger and I reflected on what Professor Vogl had said about there being a genetic component to my cancer. Perhaps this was so at other levels of inheritance too, and that these furious women needed to be heard.

Am I maybe (dare I hope) doing this not just for me, but for the ancestral line too? I have no idea, can only pray that it is all connected, and that deep healing is possible.

Well, plenty of bile was certainly being manifested!

Once I felt better it was only a couple of weeks before I was due to go back for the next treatment. Professor Vogl gave me good news of tumour shrinkage each time, but always said a bit more ablation was needed. The next one would be the sixth and hopefully final one, but I was worried I wouldn't be well enough. Vogl told me to come as planned, and that he would reduce the amount of chemo drug put in.

It made me acknowledge the 'bile' in my own life too, and how frustrations could make me critical of others, especially men. I saw it in my attitude to Chetan sometimes, when he was the last person worthy of this. It was good to have seen it though, and I knew that letting go of this deeply-rooted aspect of myself was ongoing work:

In fact Chetan had told me, some time before this and when he felt I was pressuring him about something: 'Don't you realise I've been almost on the verge of a breakdown?' I was devastated and ashamed. So much he had done for me – had I been so wrapped up in my own pain that I had not seen his?

I asked for help, and it slowly came in different ways, but I realised that the anger at men, both individuals and societal, was deep in me. I started trying to 'cure' this in the simplest of ways. Whenever I caught myself criticising and blaming I sent love towards that person instead.

My guidelines:

Know that you are a part of God, inseparable from Him and all other

> *souls in this universe.*
> *Love and forgive yourself and others.*
> *Be fearless, compassionate, kind and honourable.*
> *See blessings and feel gratitude for them.*
> *Be discerning as you keep your mind open to learning.*
> *Trust and follow your intuition.*
> *If I had to be even more succinct:*
> *Love is the key to everything.*
> *– Messages from Matthew*

The night of Obama's election as US President, while the world still awaited the result, I dreamt of great streams of light coming down to the Earth, bringing a previously unknown energy. It seemed that all of us on Earth who wished to could help nurture this new energy of which Obama's election was part. It made me feel that I could still be of use in the world, even if right now I was weak.

> *Lead a life worthy of the calling to which you have been called, with all humility and gentleness, with patience, bearing one another in love, making every effort to maintain the unity of the Spirit in the bond of peace.*
> *– Ephesians 4:1–3*

As the days of feeling not great went by I was worried about being well enough for the next treatment. And fearful that it would be as bad.

Helen gave me a healing in which I felt strong light coming into me. It initially left me tired and in some discomfort, but I carried on bringing in that light and two days later I woke up feeling very different – well! The pain had gone.

Something in my liver/abdomen area has opened up. *This* is what I can do to help with the next treatment - *keep bringing in the light.*

Acupuncture again helped too. It improved my appetite immediately, and helped me sleep.

With just a few days to go before the sixth treatment, my doctor told me I was anaemic. There are different causes of anaemia, and it would need further investigation, but might mean cancelling the treatment. I didn't want it to be postponed – or to lose our airfare.

But there was good news too. My CEA counts were down to an amazing 12.5. What a change from over 6,000 when I was first diagnosed.

To my relief my blood counts were deemed good enough for the sixth and final chemoembolisation. With a lower dose of chemo, I didn't have a severe reaction this time. The first of two laser ablations would be in just three weeks, a few days before Christmas.

Memory of a past life as a persecuted woman. I am down a dark pit, no escape. I've been left here to die. I've spoken out for what I know is right. When I die I still feel despair, that nothing will ever change. Then a powerful whirling force, going on for a long time, seems to lift painful stuff out of me. I see a densely black, velvety hole or disc. I am told that one day, maybe after many more lives, I will disappear into that blackness, and that is a truly beautiful and great teaching.

I was quite frightened about the ablation. Again, healing helped and I worked on opening myself to light and to healing, to make myself more available to the ablation, and to ease the fear. After all, laser is light.

So why shouldn't I also recover?
I am open to healing.

Ten days before the first ablation was due my mother had a

severe stroke. She was found lying on the floor, where she had clearly been all night. It was possible she had also had a heart attack. She was taken to hospital, and initially it was unclear whether she would improve or not.

I felt so sad for her. Even though she was very confused, it must have been very frightening and shocking to be so suddenly debilitated. In my own frail state there was little I could do other than send love and prayer. All the work in supporting her devolved on to Liz and Nigel. My guilt about this was not going to help. They were brilliant.

The first time I spoke to Mother on the phone she was fairly lucid. To my amazement she spontaneously remembered about my impending treatment and its importance. I was very touched, and felt her love for me.

Frankfurt old town was abuzz with a Christmas fair, full of glüwein and gingerbread stalls. It was a nice distraction from what was about to happen. The ablation followed a similar procedure to the chemoembolisation, but this time small cuts were made in the skin over the liver, and needles inserted into the liver. Disturbing, but not too painful.

I push open our garden gate. I am home. I've survived. Back to the cats, our house, our friends, and soon my second Christmas since being diagnosed with 'terminal' cancer.

> A favourite sight – orange-tipped buds on the beech trees, seen from the house against dark conifers and ablaze with early spring sunlight. I have lived to see it again.

The ablation is in my dreams. It appears in an image of something containing leaking, dirty water. The dream shows me there are choices to be made too. Is the cultured lady reminding me of what I value in life, and that I need to work with that in myself? As she pieces together precious old recipes, is she rediscovering ancient ways of living well, and healing? The man in the dream who has grown exquisite, old-fashioned roses is surely telling me that I too must 'cultivate my own garden'.

Christmas Eve. I am still here, and intend to be for many more.

Christmas is both jolly and sad. We stay with Liz and Paul, where there's a big, boisterous gathering of Paul's family. But Mum was also invited, and we raise a glass to her in hospital, where she seems to be becoming more confused. She probably doesn't know it's Christmas. Chetan has visited her, and she mistakes him for the bishop. We wonder whether to give her the presents we'd bought, or if that would just add to her pain and confusion. Perhaps we'll delay it.

I am so grateful to still be here, and for all the kindnesses shown me. Chetan gives me some healing CDs – I'm starting this next bit of the journey with some good allies.

Boxing Day. Just saw the sun starting to come up over the bank of trees. So lovely, pinky. Stood and watched it for a long time until it had risen right into the sky, letting it be part of me, filling me. As it rose above the trees it became golden, then there were intense flashes of purple within it and coming from it. I felt this was somehow connected with a prayer I had made, to understand and accept death. I can't put it into words - it was like having another part of the great mystery revealed to me, becoming part of me.

Thank you.

Going downstairs to make tea, I found that Paul's father had also watched the sun rise. Like me, he had given thanks for another day, as he said he did every day. He had faced illness, and was now seeing himself growing older. When in our lives do we start wondering how many more sunrises?

There were two other Christmas gifts from Chetan which

became of great significance. The first was a beautiful new journal, with pictures of Tibetan Buddhas on the covers and lovely big pages just waiting to be written and drawn in.

He gave me the other present when we got home, saying he hadn't wanted to give it to me when we were with the others. It was a CD called *Being with Dying*, by Roshi Joan Halifax, a Buddhist nun. Chetan thought I might be upset or even offended by such a gift, but far from it. I respected his thoughtfulness. That CD became of great importance to me, taking me into a new understanding of death and dying, and even leading me to a new friend.

We visited Mother in hospital. She was in a depressing, post-war brick unit with rows of beds lining either side of the ward. She looked so small and helpless huddled under the bedding, and didn't seem to recognise me. The staff told me not to stay long as she had an infection they were worried I might pick up. It was sad.

As the year drew to its end I noticed I was less identified with the work I had done. I no longer seemed to need to label myself as an art therapist, or indeed anything. I was just me.

Chapter 17

It was the start of another year. I certainly wasn't into making new year resolutions – unless it was just to live as long and as well as possible. Life felt too unpredictable for that. But I did want to look back at the year just gone, so that I could step cleanly into the new one.

Looking back was more painful than I'd expected.

I can hardly believe what I've come through, how I've endured it. I'd expected to look at the bad *and* good of the year, but so far it's only been possible to deal with the painful, dark stuff - the chemo up to the end of March, all the hospital visits and the ghastly prognoses, the trauma of making the decision about having the Germany treatment, the procedures themselves, let alone the fear of dying and the pain, the grief at the loss of my life as it was, and the physical symptoms.

That's how it's had to be today - looking at the dark. At least I managed to put some of it in a painting.

The early January weather was oppressive – fogbound and bitterly cold. It seemed to intensify my anger and distress at starting the new year so upset and fearful.

As I talked with Chetan about it I felt as though I had a great wound in me, going from the liver to the rectum. I instantly felt a glimmer of yet another past life. I was reluctant to look any further, to bring forth even more strong emotion, but I also knew that stifling it would be still more distressing. These past lives had arisen spontaneously several times since I had been diagnosed, and I still have no idea if they come from my personal 'history', or from a collective unconscious. But they are very vivid, playing themselves out with no conscious direction. I trust their messages and relevance.

In this one I saw myself as a very young soldier full of

excitement and bravado, shocked and horrified when he was mowed down in battle. He died of a wound snaking down from waist to groin. I saw his body being nibbled at by animals, before being taken away with many others and being given a loving family burial. It was hard for the youth to accept he had died, but healing came to him in the spirit world. Beings of light cocooned him, like swaddling a baby, and healed any trace of the trauma of the wound with light. Other beings arrived, who I felt were my spiritual family and connected with Osho, to give support too.

The healer woman spoke of acceptance. Acceptance of having had this life, this wound, this death. I knew there was a strong message there for me in my present life, as I found it hard to accept not just the cancer, but the very cycle of life and death.

> *We shall not cease from exploration*
> *And the end of all our exploring*
> *Will be to arrive where we started*
> *And know the place for the first time.*
> *– TS Eliot*

It looked as though Mother would never be able to return home. There was no way she would be able to look after herself. This was not unexpected, but very sad. And as much as anything I felt awful about Liz and Nigel having to cope with it all. I could only ask for love and support for them and her.

The second laser ablation was scheduled for mid-January. Fear again. Of pain, of the possibility that it might still not be the last one and then how we would find more money, and of the cancer starting up again.

> Winter is reluctant to go. Easter, on our favourite Cornish beach, and we push against relentless winds. But sun shines through towering turquoise waves. I too am full of extremes. Our wedding anniversary, Chetan's birthday, daffodils, long

light evenings, holding back the dread of a scan. Celandines catch brilliant sun beneath a wind-tossed gorse bush.

Before each treatment in Germany I had blood tests done here (thanks to my wonderful, supportive GP and her practice). This time they showed that the CEA levels were very slightly up. Only slightly, but anything was enough to knock me.

A few minutes after I'd heard this news by phone, my old friend Alimo called. What wonderful timing. How precious it is to just be able to share and cry with an old companion.

Alimo had come back into my life after some years of us losing contact. We had taught at the same place, and had become sannyasins of Osho (then Bhagwan Shree Rajneesh) at the same time. A warm, generous person, I had missed her in the years when we'd lost touch. She had somehow heard of my illness and managed to locate us. A real gift that came through the illness.

Know that I am held in healing light and love at all times. So much being given to me by so many, both known and unknown to me. I am so blessed just to be having this treatment. Live each moment as fully, joyfully and lovingly as possible.

Sannyasin friends came the day before we went to Germany. They brought food, and we sang and meditated together. Their love and generosity calmed me, and I was reminded to tune in to my inner being throughout the procedure.

Remember the Buddha within.

Being a sannyasin of Osho has been the most extraordinary gift in my life. Sometimes I needed to be reminded of that, and of the depths and heights to which it has taken me.

I am lying on the operating couch in Frankfurt University Hospital. It's the second ablation. Cuts are made in my abdomen for the needles to be inserted. I've been sedated and am quite drowsy. I must have fallen asleep, for I come to with a scream of pain, thinking the procedure is over and trying to back my body away from the pain in my abdomen. A nurse angrily tells me that they haven't started the procedure, and that if I don't calm down they will have to stop, and I will go home without it being done. I'm almost hysterical, and even more frightened once I realise they haven't even begun. I try to calm myself, but it's difficult. I think they must have given me more sedative, because thankfully I do calm down.

Strangely I have less pain after this ablation than after the first one.

Next day we are as usual in Professor Vogl's elegant waiting room. Good modern paintings on the walls, gifts from patients in the cabinets. We tentatively chat with other patients, wanting to know what has helped them but perhaps wary of any greater intimacy.

Vogl tells me that they weren't able to remove every bit of tumour from the liver. He wants to check me with a CT scan in two months, rather than the expected three. He also describes the colon tumour as a 'time bomb' which could activate at any time. He now thinks I shouldn't have it operated on as it's such a major op and my immune system is low, so it could spread.

I'm left feeling in a different place from what I had expected. Maybe the cancer is going to start up again sooner than I'd expected. Oh God.

> A few sneezes, a tickle in the throat. Instant fear. If a cold comes, will it turn to pneumonia, will it bring my death?

As for the op, which I had hoped might be possible by the end of this treatment, I have mixed feelings. There is some relief that, if I take Vogl's advice, I don't have to go chasing around trying to find someone in the UK who will agree to do it, and to have such a major procedure. But underneath that I feel desolate. So it's hopeless then. It's hard to bear.

So now I think it's about finding that equanimity between believing I can still heal, live with this for a long time, and accepting that I could die a lot sooner.

I just heard a bird singing outside, so beautifully. Even though it's still not really light. There is so much beauty in the world.

Travelling back home we once again stayed with Jonathan and Fran, and our distress was calmed by their friendship. Our room had been made so welcoming, there was lovely food, there was feeling cared for, part of life.

Mother was taken from hospital to a home near Liz, where I hoped she would be able to live out this last part of her life in as fulfilling a way as possible. I also hoped it would not be too unbearable and gruelling for my siblings.

Back home, early February. Professor Vogl was going to want to check me again around late March. Surely we didn't need to go to Germany for a scan? We decided to approach Dr Daniel in Plymouth to see if I could have a scan in the UK, and send the results on to Germany. If this was possible it would save a tiring journey, and a lot of money.

I was still adjusting to my new life as a person with cancer. Painful dreams would remind me that I was no longer working with old colleagues, or that I couldn't take part in a yoga class because I was too ill, I was 'different'. I veered between knowing the love of friends, and feeling like an outsider.

Don't surrender your loneliness
So quickly.
Let it cut more deep.
Let it ferment and season you
As few human

Or even divine ingredients can.
Something missing in my heart tonight
Has made my eyes so soft,
My voice so tender,
My need of God
Absolutely
Clear.
– Absolutely Clear: Hafiz

Chapter 18

However much I hope to heal, I am dying. It might be later, it might be sooner, but it is so. Of course, it is so for us all. It's hard to believe, despite all the evidence.

The *Being with Dying* CD was making me really face up to my death. Yet I found it a relief, and listened to it for days on end during my after-lunch rest. I heard about Roshi Joan Halifax's work with people facing death, but above all about the Buddhist attitude to dying. Here was the relief – that death was seen as something of immense importance, to be entered into with as much consciousness as possible. And there were practices which could help with this. There was great compassion too, and a sense that here was a body of knowledge and insight gleaned over thousands of years which is still – perhaps even more so now – of immense value.

Through more fully facing dying, I was starting to look at how I might befriend it. There was just a glimmer that perhaps there was richness and learning in it, not just darkness and fear.

I looked up Roshi Joan on the Internet, and discovered that she lives in a Buddhist community in New Mexico, but sometimes gives workshops in Europe. Perhaps I could do one. I contacted the community, and to my delight got an email from her, saying that she was unlikely to be in Europe for some time, but that one of her colleagues was soon returning to the UK to live. Her name was Jean, and Roshi would pass my name on to her. It's hard to explain how precious that felt – to reach out and ask for help, and find it so very fully met.

May I be at peace
As I live and as I die.
May all beings be at peace
As they live and as they die.
– Loving Kindness meditation

Meanwhile Chetan and I had decided to try to get a scan done in Devon, and in effect to get back into the NHS system. Another nightmare ensued. There was no available appointment with Dr Daniel for weeks, and Professor Vogl had said I should be scanned within two months. Chetan was brilliant, phoning secretaries, and getting help from the hospital's patient liaison. Not that it did much good in the end.

It looked quite promising at one stage. Through Chetan's persistence we got a last-minute cancelled appointment. But I was astonished to discover that they still didn't have my notes from the previous hospital – five months after having been referred, so I wasn't really part of their system. So no scan. It all felt very rushed, back to being a statistic again, whilst at the same time there being no sense from the Plymouth hospital of urgency about my scan. There was no possibility of one for weeks, then Dr Daniel would be away, so the earliest I could get any scan results was mid-May. A bit different from the end of March, given how quickly Vogl had said the tumours could grow.

I wasn't happy. We looked at having the scan doing privately. Scandalously, to my way of thinking, this could be done almost immediately – but *privately* – on the very NHS scanner that was booked up for weeks. Here indeed was the two-tier system. But the cost of having it done privately was about the same as going to Germany. It felt safer and less complicated to travel to Germany for it.

The NHS is a wonderful thing, but it seems to have become so vast and institutionalised that in some places there is little room for ambitious new thinking. It's a great jewel, but needs a good deal of repolishing in places. To mix metaphors, some blinkers need to be removed so that entrenched thinking is questioned, not blindly adhered to.

We've had massive amounts of snow here for days – up to your knees everywhere. Last night when I came to bed the full moon was shining on this great expanse of white, casting shadows from the trees across the white garden. So beautiful. Then reading in bed with Chet - felt like a lovely space, knowing there was the snow outside and feeling the warmth of being there with him. Then suddenly, just like a bolt from nowhere, a huge wave of grief - how much longer will I enjoy such things, would I still be doing this in a year. Quite took my breath away.

Have to accept the grief, the fear. But I know too that I want to be more and more in a different relationship with dying, with death, as much as possible. Accepting, maybe even welcoming it, seeing it as a liberation, and an expansion of the soul.

But to live well, fully, lovingly, consciously first.

Another medicine wheel workshop. Back with a group of women who share their souls, their dreams, their lives. We build an altar in the middle of the room, honouring the many aspects of the wheel, of the world on all levels. We make little pouches of tobacco, they become sacred as we honour the tobacco, the cloth, the making, and fill them with intent. We give thanks to Great Spirit, to Grandmother Earth, Grandfather Sun, the ancestors, the dream of how we wish our world to be.

For me there are reminders of the earth mother goddess with whom I so urgently needed to make contact again in the early days of my diagnosis. Not always an easy energy – one day we will all return to her black, fertile earth, before we receive new life from her and live again.

> *As goddess of the soul, Gaia reminds us that the soul develops in dark places and that ultimately soul must be rooted in body, in earth. She is a reminder that we must ground ourselves in the reality of nature and incorporate all sides of ourselves, be they pleasant or unpleasant, light or dark.*
> *– Goddess cards*

My three tobacco pouches contain first what I need to remember: *where I come from*; then what I need to discover: *how to love life, both in this body and out of it, both life and death*; and lastly what I need to manifest: *trust, and giving thanks to the Divine*.

Amidst my work on dying, Mother's condition, and the difficulties I was facing with illness and treatment, being part of a group of women who reach out to each other, and to the divine within all things, is an affirmation of the richness of life's journey, even in times of pain.

Mother was having lots of falls in the residential home and it was now totally clear that she was never going to return to her own house. It was putting a huge burden on both Liz, who lived near to the home and visited often, and on Nigel who was taking care of financial matters and visiting frequently too.

Nigel, Liz, Chetan and I spend a weekend clearing Mother's house, so that it can be rented out to pay her nursing home fees. I had dreaded it, but it isn't as bad as I had expected. There is joy in being together in the task, knowing how hard it may be for each of us, and being kind and supportive of each other. It is a strange experience too; it's as though we are clearing out the house of someone who has died, yet Mother is still alive.

I try to honour what we are doing. I give thanks for my parents' lives, and seek to see sorting their familiar possessions as the river moving on. Every so often I am aware of a wrench in letting go of some small but familiar object. Sometimes too there is desire to keep something, but mostly I don't want much – what use would it be to me, if I do not have long to live? I am grateful though that Liz and Nigel take most of the very personal things like photos, as they both have children to whom they can be passed on. I would have struggled to know what to do with these family memories, and not been ready to let go.

Slowly the house loses its lived-in look as we sort the stuff of two lifetimes. Light patches on the walls show where Father's paintings hung for years.

We spend the night there, my last one in that house. I dream of Osho, sitting at his feet as he reminds me to 'be here now'.

The tabby cat rolls on warm spring grass. Daffodils have come again.

Before leaving I visit the oak tree in the park opposite where Father's ashes are buried. I thank him for our lives together, so much that he gave me. What has happened to him now, I wonder. He was always so sure there was nothing beyond this life. Well, one of us must be wrong! Sometimes, of course, I doubt and am cynical about anything esoteric, but at other times I just know he's around.

Then to Liz's for a few days, so that I could visit Mother in the home. It was sad to see her so bruised after more falls, and how she sometimes looked like a lost child. Very confused, but knew us both. Liz was great with her – loving and reassuring. I took her some of her favourite cake, which seemed much more meaningful than the Christmas present I had kept for her.

Again I dreamt of Osho. We were speaking on the phone! He was telling me that a woman I knew was doing well, going in the right direction. I could only hope that was me!

When you stay with the idea that you are not the body nor the mind, not even their witness but altogether beyond, your mind will grow in clarity, your desires in purity, your actions in charity and that inner distillation will take you to another world. A world of truth and fearless love.
– Nisargadatta Maharaj

This quote was sent to me by my friend Jitindriya, with whom I spoke regularly on the phone. The way she had dealt with having MS was and is a constant inspiration to me, and this quote summed up her attitude. Her friendship has become precious to me, even though we usually have to just chat on the phone. She reassures and comforts me, lets me moan, complain, be fearful. It's stuff she has had to deal with, and receives with humour and acceptance. As I've struggled to let go of all the 'doing', and relax, she tells me of the joy of resting, of being with one's self. I know there are hard times for her, and for her husband Narayano who is so supportive, but she's always there to give me a lift, remind me I'm loved, that I'm human.

The trip to Frankfurt for a CT scan was arranged. It would be at the end of March, as Vogl had suggested.

The local news ran a story of a woman who was also going to Vogl for treatment, and who attended Plymouth hospital too. She had mesothelioma, a type of lung cancer, and I was interested to know her story.

We met at a little café on the edge of Dartmoor. It was hard to believe that this lively, vibrant woman was deemed terminally ill. But then I found it hard to believe of myself too. Debbie told us that she had been getting very good results from Vogl's treatment, apparently surprising the UK oncologists who had been pretty sceptical about it.

Debbie was funding her treatment with compensation she had received for contracting the disease. Her father had worked in Plymouth docks, and came home every night with his clothes covered in asbestos, in the days before its dangers were known. Her 'compensation' was pretty small, but enough to buy some treatment – and some hope.

Debbie told me that the actress Farrah Fawcett had also had treatment from Vogl, for anal cancer. She had since died, but it seemed likely that this had extended her life.

Around this time I noticed a sense of shame in me.

I felt ashamed of having cancer.

Why hadn't I been able to prevent it, or to recognise it? Had I somehow brought it about, allowed it? Did it mean, particularly because of where it was located, that I was full of shit?

This sense of shame, and by extension of guilt, is ultimately not helpful. I do think that stresses in life are contributory factors, but there are many other factors too – environmental, genetic, and many others. I found it helpful to look at the stresses there had been in my life in the couple of years preceding diagnosis, and hope that I have learnt from them. But carrying guilt, and shame, is not helpful or healing. I have tried to let go of my shame at having let my human frailty be made so visible.

Chetan and I are on an ancestors workshop. We are looking at how people may die feeling incomplete in this life in some way, how this might affect their ability to move on after they have left their body, and if help can be given to them to do so. I make contact with a great aunt on my father's side who died of breast cancer and seems to have felt very alone. Perhaps another raging woman, but this one feels more sad and lonely than the bitter ones on my mother's side. Her fear and sense of isolation have made it difficult for her to leave the earth plane, and I ask that she may be taken towards the light by other loving ancestors, to be loved and acknowledged, and find peace.

I feel now that some part of our soul 'visits' the earth in the physical body, where we may meet up again with particular other beings, and after death we return 'home' - to the greater soul, the spirit, where healing and cleansing happen. There we are on some level reunited with loved ones, or encounter other souls and beings who are our wider spiritual family. In this life we can also learn to acknowledge or accept the difficult, shadow parts of our beings.

Strange stuff. But it feels very real. From other participants we hear many touching stories, and it expands my understanding of what may happen after death. After leaving the body the soul may sometimes get ensnared on its journey, especially if there is trauma or fear at the time of bodily death. Help from the earthly or spiritual realms may assist these beings to accept they are dead, that it is time to move on, and safe to do so. If this is so, it must make the care of the dying even more important.

> From high above it the river looks like an unmoving silver chain. Upstream, our home. Downstream, rock where one day my ashes will lie beneath Dartmoor soil. But now, children play beside the river in soft spring sunlight.

Chapter 19

Just a couple of weeks before the scan in Germany, and I swung between extremes of feelings, joy in the moment and fear of what lay ahead.

Sitting outside in the early morning. A low mist down by the river, soft sunshine. I feel the incredible beauty of it, also my grief.

Yesterday saw on a bloods report that my CEA levels have gone up again, so the cancer must be more active again since the chemoembolisation finished in November.

Suddenly changed from feeling full of hope and good energy to hopeless, that all is downhill from now on. But trying to hold on to my centre too, to that part of me which I know never dies.

For a while I was alright, but then a tiny thing, an ordinary action of putting something away in a drawer, just triggered me. It seemed so precious. All those everyday little things of life, the things I take for granted, they are all part of my life, and this small, everyday act suddenly represented all I will one day lose.

Sitting here now I see the drops of water on the tree, catching the light, Sophie sitting beside me, the mist rising slowly over the green, five jackdaws flying past. I know my beloved Chetan is upstairs in bed, and has just held me and hugged me. It is all so precious, so delicate, so hard to let go of.

I must draw on all I have learned and experienced. If the cancer is reactivating - oh god, it's hard, but I want to be present, courageous, loving, accepting, *but* also living in hope and in vibrant energy.

I pray for energy. For love.

Yet my energy levels were really good. Being off chemo was great. My cells were jumping up and down in delight.

There was a lovely weekend with old friends Pete and Jane, in Wales. I was still excited to be out anywhere much, and crossing the Severn Bridge was a feast for the eyes. As indeed were Jane's wonderful puddings for the stomach! I felt humbled by their open-hearted generosity. We walked round the lovely new Cardiff waterfront, and felt spring arriving from the top of a mountain.

> Two cuckoos are calling across our valley. It is Beltane, the buds bursting. I have so much to celebrate.

In a healing session with Helen, some words came to her spontaneously. I knew I would find them helpful as I faced the trip to Germany. 'You have always been walking in the light,' she said, 'whether you were spirit in body or spirit alone. Your journey has been long (many lives) and fruitful.'

That's what I needed to remember. That I was more than just the physical body, or even my mind and feelings. It helped.

I sat in a field full of daffodils, and thought I would never stop crying. Later I drew an image of what I wanted for the year ahead, and daffodils emerging from dark, black soil appeared on the paper. That was my vision: that out of this dark underground place could come a blossoming of light and colour.

My prayers for this year:

May I have the awareness to return to my centre, my consciousness

May I be grateful for all I have in my life

May I share love, give and receive love - and laugh.

It's this strange balance all the time - to love and to live fully every moment, whilst also accepting and being ready to let go and die.

There are new tumours in the liver. Four of them, says Professor Vogl. And possibly some in the lungs.

I've been expecting something, but not this bad. I reel out of the hospital in a daze, Chetan holding my hand so tightly. We walk along the side of the river where a sprinkling of slushy snow still lies.

Vogl has told me that I should now look for systemic chemo, to stop the spread that is obviously happening. There is nothing more that he can do at present. He suggests further chemotherapy, or possibly a drug called Avastin.

I know, though, that the treatment has not been a failure. It has dealt with such a lot of the tumours. I have no doubt that it has given me more time. But what now?

We have time to spend before the flight home, and wander around a splendid art gallery containing pictures by German old masters. Is this what I want to be doing with my precious time? Yes, it is, to see beauty and creativity, and remember people whose lives have been lived that way. Walking back to the hotel we pass through long archways of trees. They were beautiful in summer, their softly rustling leaves giving shade on the dusty path. Now their bare, gnarled branches form eerie Gothic shapes beneath the street lights. Everything changes.

But they're still trees. I'm still me. Oh yes, and the geese are still there. We glimpse them sitting in the girders beneath a bridge, away from the cold water.

> As if in one day the moor is full of new life. A foal, wet and glistening, minutes old. Violets studding the path, lambs bouncing across the road. A heron, motionless in fast-flowing water.

I wonder if I can even face more chemo.

As soon as we got back home we tried to get an appointment with Dr Daniel at Plymouth as soon as possible. He couldn't see me for nearly three weeks, which for me seemed like an absolute age. Was it urgent or not? Presumably this new growth had been happening for at least a couple of months, so it certainly felt urgent to me. I found it very upsetting. Chetan and Liz started doing all they could to get an earlier appointment with him.

But I did already have a private appointment with Dr Rosy Daniel booked for a few days' time. I hoped that with her I could look at whether I actually did want more chemo. My body had gone through so much, I wasn't sure if I could face it. Perhaps she could advise me on what alternative treatments might at least support me.

This is what I have to do now. Return to the centre, my core, so that I am not buffeted by all the emotions, the events, the decisions.

Become the watcher, always from that centred place.

Over the next few days there were so many 'chance' meetings with old friends, and a day full of others phoning me, their support holding me steady.

And soon after our sad return from Germany there were things to celebrate. It was our first wedding anniversary, and I was determined to put aside the grief and fear, and enjoy a day of love and gratitude with Chetan. We had hoped to be away in our little caravan for a few days, but it was just not possible with all the chasing of hospital appointments. So we journeyed to St Ives for just a day, and a wonderful and special time it was.

This is hard to write, but I realise our first wedding anniversary may also be our last one. This cancer seems so serious now. It is hard to believe. But for today may I give thanks.

There was lunch in a little beachside restaurant, the cold wind making huge white waves, tea in the Tate and a drive down the fabulous coast to Zennor for a drink in the Tinners Arms. Many times I dipped into thoughts of my condition, the sorrow that I might never be there again, but it was full of joy, fun and celebration too.

Driving back home I watched an extraordinary moon. It was a strange shape, with one or two huge rays of light coming from it. Perhaps it was a partial eclipse. I have always loved the moon, even writing a book about it once, and I felt that it was now giving me a message. Change and the unknown are beautiful too.

> *Freedom from attachment is freedom from death. Freedom from attachment is freedom from the wheel of birth and death. Freedom from attachment makes you capable of entering into the universal light and becoming one with it. And that is the greatest blessing, the ultimate ecstasy beyond which nothing else exists. You have come home.*
> *– Osho*

Chapter 20

Two days later, the second celebration. And the start of one of the most intense times in my life.

It was Chetan's birthday. That was the celebration, but that very morning we'd been phoned with a last-minute appointment to see Dr Daniel at Plymouth. I was grateful for it, but scared, and guilty too for Chetan having to spend his birthday this way.

It was my third time at this hospital, but I had still never received any treatment there. Strange.

By the time I get to the appointment I am really starting to think I can't face any more treatment. Dr Daniel is kind and thorough. He goes through all the treatment I've had in Germany. I tell him what Professor Vogl has said about now needing systemic chemo. I then have to list all the chemo drugs I've taken recently. There are quite a lot – as well as the Oxalyplatin from the first six months of chemo there's capecitabin almost constantly, plus a cocktail of other chemo drugs delivered direct into the liver during the chemoembolisation.

I've had enough, Dr Daniel tells me, I can't have more. He presents me with statistics of how various drugs would prolong my life by a month or so, but at a huge price to my well-being. In fact, he says, the bowel cancer drugs would have little effect, as I would have developed a kind of resistance to them.

So no more medical treatment. Actually I felt relieved, that the decision I'd already been considering was anyway the only option. I'm amazed at how calm I felt, and quite strong.

I don't know what I would have felt or wanted if he had offered me treatment. Probably I would have leapt at it. I just don't know. But it had turned out that he wasn't going to offer me any such option. He was unequivocal about it.

All he offered me was a referral to a palliative care consultant.

'You're a brave woman,' he said. I didn't feel it. Just stunned.

As we drove away from the hospital I kept trying to bring myself back to my centre. To not freak out seemed all-important. I'd just been told I was only fit for palliative care – I was dying – but I was determined to stay as still, calm and aware as I could. It was as though a channel of light ran through me from head to toe, through the centre of my body, and that's where I had to stay.

'Don't go hunting for anything else,' Dr Daniel had said. He was encouraging me to stay calm I guess, to take this on board.

But it was Chetan's birthday. In a daze we headed in the direction of the coast for a walk by the sea. We drove past a National Trust property and just decided to drop in for a cup of tea before travelling further.

Still dazed, I could hardly believe it when I saw two old friends. They were miles from their home, and this was a place we never visited ourselves. I can only think the gods were with us yet again.

We sat with Ute – an old friend from Bristol Cancer Help Centre days – and David, eating brownies, sharing the devastating news, celebrating Chetan's birthday, hearing news of their grandchildren, crying and enjoying being together. Just life! I could not have asked for more at that moment.

Afterwards, standing by the sea at Hope Cove. Sunny early evening, together. I later wrote in my journal that it would probably be the last time I was with Chetan for his birthday.

This is the hardest part. Letting go of the people I love. Maybe it is only letting go of them in these bodies, this life. But it's still quite unbelievable that it must happen, and so painful. But that's what *will* happen one day. Just love them, love them, love them right now so there are no regrets.

Telling Liz and Nigel what Dr Daniel had said was hard, but they were wonderful. I felt guilty at the pain they were having to endure, particularly with Mother being so ill. It seemed to me that the best I could do was to show them that I was all right as much as I could.

Now this part of my life is to live in as happy, peaceful, aware and loving a way as I can.

Mercifully it sounds as though the dying process need not be painful - with the liver there's usually not too much pain, and it can be controlled. Mostly will be getting more tired and weaker. This is hard to write, but I know I have so many loving helpers and guides and supporters, physical and spiritual, alongside me.

The appointment, made ages before with Dr Rosy Daniel, just happened to be for the very next day. I wondered if it was still worth going as I'd just been told nothing more could be done. But I thought Rosy would be able to advise me on supplements and anything that would help me stay well as long as possible, so it would be worth the journey to Bath.

I recalled the words from the other Dr Daniel, to not go seeking anything else. Maybe he was encouraging me to relax and be calm. But I wasn't quite ready to just sit back and do nothing.

It was also twenty-five years to the day since my then partner Andrew had died of leukaemia. I sent him love and blessings, and hoped I could get through the day being as centred as possible amidst all this intensity.

Now another day, another moment. Live it with joy.

Liz meets us in Bath. She has generously made it possible to come at the last minute. I feel heartbroken when we meet, so sad at what I am putting everyone through, but buoyed up by her love and vitality. I feel proud of her, what she's achieved in her life. We sit in a gorgeous café, eating wonderful food and talking about my death.

Rosy is extraordinary. She scoops us up into her caring and expertise. She seems to take my situation totally in her stride, and comes up with several suggestions that just might help me. I'm totally amazed that she has further options to consider.

So much for my promise to the other Dr Daniel to not consider any other treatments!

Rosy encouragingly tells me of Penny Brohn, co-founder of Bristol Cancer Help Centre (now of course called after Penny). Having had breast cancer for many years, Penny was referred to a hospice when it had spread to her spine. In great pain, she was told that she only had a very short time to live. Rosy urged a surgeon to see her, her spine was operated on and she lived more than another four years.

And again, Rosy says that the liver is the priority.

> We shiver in the village hall where we meet to meditate. But there are homemade jams and new-laid eggs for sale, and someone has baked a cake to share. Little jewels, vast spaces.

Rosy's most promising suggestion is to contact Dr Alice Gillams at University College Hospital London again. Dr Gillams had suggested that my case for radio frequency ablation might be looked at again in a year's time. It is about a year since then. But, Rosy advises, I should seek a private appointment. It will take too long to go through the NHS system of referrals and appointment lists – I need to move fast.

I'm excited, but doubtful too. Quite apart from whether Dr Gillams would take me on, would there be any point in having another ablation? Would it just be Canute holding the tide at bay? Yet if there's a moral to Canute's story it's that even the mightiest of us are humble before the forces of nature, we just do what we can. And doing what I could at least now contained some other possibilities.

Saying goodbye to Liz is both painful and joyful. We're venturing into yet more unknown territory.

On the way home we call in on Jonathan and Fran. I feel blessed by their friendship and love. They invite us to come soon for a few days, which I know will be so good.

What can I do for Liz? Just show her I'm ok, happy (when I am) and share with her. I'm so happy that she and Chet have a lot of love and respect for each other, and can share all of this - and I can also know that when I die they will be supporting and loving each other.

The counselling sessions with Jen had been so useful, and I was due to see her soon after the trip to Bath. Great timing, after those few days. The session was good. To my surprise I was quite accepting and calm. But was I just resigning myself to dying quite soon, I wondered. No, it was more about looking at things in my life which I felt I had resolved and dealt with.

I wanted to go into whatever lay ahead in as calm and accepting a way as possible.

I sit watching a patch of bare earth. It's good just sitting there, looking, feeling the sun. I have planted this year's vegetable seeds.

Chapter 21

Years ago I worked in London at the *Radio Times* in Marylebone High Street. It's just a short distance from Harley Street and I would sometimes see people going into the smart clinics. I would wonder about their stories. I never saw myself being one of those patients.

But here I am, in Harley Street with Liz. Another visit to an old, and as I thought finished, part of my life. We pass familiar streets, even some of the same shops. It reminds me that working in the buzz of London had been exciting. But a few ghosts are still knocking around too, and it is a good chance for them to jump up and down a bit and then be laid to rest. A difficult relationship, a time of uncertainty about where I was going in my life after living in an Osho community for several years, the struggle of commuting, decisions about having children… they are all there, just waiting to be released into the spring air.

This time I'm here to see Dr Gillams. A Harley Street clinic is rather different from an NHS one. Thick carpets, comfy chairs and a low, discreet buzz of conversation. But the people waiting here look no less drawn with anxiety than those I've seen in shabbier NHS waiting rooms.

Dr Gillams, a pioneer in radio frequency ablation, gives me an ultrasound scan. I truly expect her to say there is nothing she can do for me. She can treat me, she says. I'm overwhelmed with astonishment and gratitude.

I need to know if it's worth it. She assures me that though it's not a cure, it should give me many more months of life than I would otherwise have. We talk about the preciousness of that. The treatment will be soon, in this clinic. And it will cost thousands – again. I'm not even sure at the moment if we can find any more money.

There's more. Dr Gillams suggests that I ask for a referral to the NHS hospital in which she works, University College

Hospital London. That way I should be able to get on a list for ablation, ready for the next time I need it. But I do need this one promptly, she suggests, rather than waiting to get on that list.

Dr Gillams also says that by getting a referral to UCH I'll be able to see an oncologist there. When I tell her I've been told I can't have more chemo she says it's still worth a try. There could be other treatment possibilities, and clinical trials are often happening at UCH as it's a London teaching hospital. I'm even more overwhelmed, though daren't raise my hopes too much.

I *can* have radio frequency ablation. Initially I felt quite numb, shocked - I'd gone so deeply into accepting I only had a much shorter time that it was quite hard to step out of that again. What an incredible thing. Now just have to find the money for it.

Liz and I go for lunch in Marylebone High Street, stunned by what we've been told. Office workers scurry back to their work at 2. I'm glad I left that way of life many years ago. This is like a different life now – and I'm still in it!

> Yesterday picnickers splashed in the river, today the cuckoo calls again. Primroses are giving way to buttercups. I sit amidst beauty.

Back home that night I lie in the bath, sobbing. Even though Dr Gillams has offered me more than I'd ever hoped for, I'm just wrung out. I feel like a little baby, exhausted from crying, needing to be bathed and soothed. Chetan washes me; I am infantile.

It was good to be home. Over the weekend I sat in the sunny spring garden, talked with many friends on the phone – Atosh, Pete, Alimo, Maya, Jitindriya, Nigel, Liz. They fed me, built me back up. Chetan gave me a healing. I grew calmer.

Dr Gillams had explained that the RFA would be done under

general anaesthetic, but that I would only be in the clinic one night. (Just as well, I thought, given how much a night in Harley Street must cost.) During the procedure the stomach would be displaced in order to get to the liver. There was likely to be some pain for about two weeks afterwards. My poor body. I needed to start 'talking' to it, explaining it will be ok.

> The cat brings in a dying mouse. I see it take its last breath, and am ridiculously upset. Bright eyes, soft fur, perfect. I bury it under leaves beneath a hedge.

I needed the treatment soon, but there were two problems.

The first was finding the money. We'd exhausted my little pots of pension, and gifts from generous friends and family. Mercifully, Chetan was able to access funds from a will which would have eventually come to us. I gave thanks to his deceased parents for all they were still doing for us. I was so lucky.

Chetan dealing with my pensions had released some funds, though at what cost to him I couldn't know. I did know they asked awful questions about how long I might live. I'd never wanted to know my prognosis, but they certainly wouldn't have released the money if they'd considered me anything other than imminently terminal.

The other concern with the RFA was potentially a much nicer one. Ever since I'd been diagnosed we'd been dreaming of a good holiday abroad, just relaxing somewhere warm. Recently it had finally looked possible, I was well enough to travel. So we had booked two weeks on Kefalonia for the end of April, as we'd always loved Greece. We'd found a cheap deal and, amazingly, had been given a substantial gift from the anonymous friend of a friend to help us. We really didn't want to miss going, but it looked as though the RFA might be just a week before – would I be well enough?

So today, waiting to hear when I can have the procedure. Stay centred, calm, positive.

Know that I AM ALIVE AND LIVING right up to the very end.

I AM ALIVE. I AM LIVING.

Thank you God. Please show me how to live well and fully. To be of service in whatever way I can be. To live in the light. To love. To give and receive. To live consciously in the wonder of being alive.

I didn't have to wait long to hear. So that I could go away, they would do the ablation in just two days' time.

I woke on the morning of the procedure with dread and fear, but knowing that I could find courage, and that this gift was one of more life. It was time to truly love being in life, to discover what else I needed to do, to love. I had dreamt of a lovely young woman living with her wealthy merchant father. One day a dishevelled old man, returning from abroad, had come with a letter addressed to her in writing she did not know. She was unable to read it at the time, but knew it would ultimately change her life, for the better. I wondered if the ablation was going to be a new beginning, a change in my life, too.

On the day I die, when I'm being
Carried toward the grave, don't weep.
Don't say 'He's gone! He's gone!'
Death has nothing to do with going away.
The sun sets and the moon sets,
But they're not gone. Death
Is a coming together.
The tomb looks like a prison,
But it's really a release
Into Union.
The human seed goes down into the ground
Like a bucket into the well where Joseph is.
It grows and comes up full

Of some unimagined beauty.
Your mouth closes here.
And immediately opens
With a shout of joy there.
– Rumi

It felt like a hotel, but it was a clinic in Harley Street. I was about to have the ablation whilst almost feeling on holiday. But that soon passed as I was visited by nurses and anaesthetists for tests.

The procedure went well. I awoke in some discomfort, nothing too bad. Chetan was there when I came to, which was so reassuring. Later Nigel came from work to visit me. I hadn't often seen him in a business suit. I hope I remembered to tell him how nice he looked. I felt grateful for the bonds of love between us of which I had become much more aware since my illness, and for his great kindness.

The treatment was similar to the ablations I had had in Germany, but the 'burning' was done through radio frequency rather than laser.

I was discharged next morning after a CT scan, out into the bright, busy street. Chetan took me to Liz's, where I was to stay a few days until I felt up to the journey back to Devon. Things would soon settle down, I thought. There was pain, but it was bearable, and I knew I'd gradually feel less groggy.

Life seemed set to keep coming up with new challenges. On the third day after the treatment Mother was taken into hospital with double pneumonia.

She might be dying. There was no way of knowing whether she would respond to the antibiotics and recover. But even if she did, 'recovery' was never going to mean getting over the huge damage from the stroke. She had become more and more confused and disorientated, often not recognising us. Painful to see, and we could only speculate on how distressed she was in the parallel world she seemed to have entered. I think all of us wondered whether or not we should hope for her recovery.

I could not visit her. I was in pain, and my immune system was likely to be still very low so going to a hospital seemed impossible, certainly very unwise. Liz and Nigel were shining stars in coping with it and being with her.

I have to hand it over to Liz and Nigel. I am trying to 'hold' her from here, asking that she be supported and given what she needs, if she is dying now or not.

Life feels so strange. So uncertain and unknown.

The day after Mum was taken into hospital was Easter Day. I woke feeling sad – about her being in hospital, about Easters past and the possibility – or not – of future ones.

Within minutes of me waking Chetan phoned. Our sannyasin friend Neera had died that morning. Actually the way he put it was that she had 'left the body', and I felt the truth of that rather than of 'dying' and its implication that nothing of her remained. What a vibrant, feisty woman she was. I sent her prayers, and asked that she be helped through this transition.

I know all is merciful and loving.

I had a few more days with Liz's family, enjoying my two lively nephews, Liz's cheerful and uplifting support, chats with Paul. By the time I was fit to go home it was still not clear what was happening with Mother. She seemed to be responding to antibiotics, but wasn't out of the woods. Liz was due to go on a long-planned birthday weekend to Barcelona. She really needed that break after all she'd had to deal with. I just hoped it would be possible.

Chapter 22

I'm back home, awake after a really good night's sleep. Still needed painkillers, and woke a bit in the night with deep sweats, but I'd fallen asleep listening to the gentling sound of *The Messiah*, live on the radio.

I've woken up calm, peaceful, happy. I got up to make drinks, and saw that in the garden a mass of primroses have come up. Then I felt a bit faint, must have overdone it. Chetan just held me for ages, it was so beautiful. I know how extraordinarily blessed I am.

And look - porridge has arrived now!

Perhaps there is always a shadow to every light. A few nights later I had a painful dream in which I became aware of an awful, destructive force coming towards the two of us as we lay in bed. There was no escape, and I knew this force would break everything apart, like treading on an egg. I felt terrified. And there was little comfort in waking from the dream, because there is indeed no escape from death.

Life kept on putting this in front of my face. We went to a celebration for Neera, prior to her cremation. A village hall was filled with huge boughs of blossoming magnolia, pictures of Neera. Her musician friends played music from Osho's ashram, we cried, laughed, danced, hugged.

I had been fine at the celebration, but woke next morning feeling desperately sad.

I don't want to die. I don't want to leave all that is so precious to me - my life, Chet, all my beloved ones, even the cats, my paintings, the house. I felt absolutely desolate. Chetan held me, just allowed me the space to cry and cry. I'm calmer now, but still sad, and very tired.

Those who wanted to were invited that morning to view Neera's body before it was cremated. She looked so small, in a wicker casket as though she was being cradled like a baby. There were flowers around her, and in her hand. It seemed so important to honour her, give thanks for her vibrant life.

But there was delight too. It was Liz's birthday and she had been able to go to Barcelona, as Mother's condition had stabilised though she was still in hospital. I wished my dear sister a wonderful day, full of sunshine and fun.

Another difficult dream. Chetan was telling me I had to leave him for a while, and he would be with a different woman. I saw her - she was strong and vibrant, with fat legs! She was looking through a wall to something on the other side. I felt so jealous, and so angry that I couldn't be with him - violent and helpless, and knew that I just had to go off by myself.

I know this is about dying, about leaving Chet which is surely one of the most difficult things. The woman was life - he'd be engaging with her, and she was able to see through the wall to whatever lies ahead. I had no choice but to go. But at least in the dream it was a temporary state - I would be back with him one day, so maybe that has taken root within me - that everything changes, moves, and love is always there.

Although I felt clear that the woman in the dream represented Chetan's life without me in it, it could of course also have been about the possibility of him being with someone else after my death. It may seem strange but we have rarely touched on how his life might be then. If he ever does want to broach it, that's fine, but I want to respect the fact that it will be *his* life, not mine with him. He may not have any idea what he will do, because that will be another time. Whatever it is, I want him to know that I totally support him in any choices he makes. I just wish him happiness and peace.

I had heard from Jean Wilkins, Roshi Joan Halifax's friend. A Tibetan Buddhist, Jean had just returned to the UK from the community in New Mexico, and was in Devon. She invited us to meet with her at Gaia House, a Buddhist retreat centre.

I liked her straight away. Chetan, Jean and I chatted over tea, and it was as though I'd known her a long time. We talked of all that had happened since my diagnosis, and Jean listened with such understanding. I knew she had experienced people dying, being alongside them through their illness and death, just by the way she responded without fear or drama. We spoke a little of meditation, of what I hoped might help me now, of facing death.

Jean's friendship has been a wonderful gift. She is unwavering in her ability to absorb my despair, my fears – and to laugh and have fun too. Whatever angel guided her here, thank you!

A few days after meeting her a book arrived from Jean. It was the full version of Roshi Joan's *Being with Dying*. It would be in my suitcase for Kefalonia.

It's bedtime, but I need to write down what a beautiful day it's been, the most exquisite spring day with sunshine, soft breeze, all the tree buds bursting with vitality. You just want to eat them. This beautiful day, when I've also felt much more energetic, is also a lesson in not holding on. It's so superb that I want it to be endless, but of course it isn't. So now I give thanks for it, move into sleep and whatever the next moment brings.

It was only a week until Chetan and I should be going on our longed-for holiday. I was steadily feeling better, and was sure I'd be able to cope with going. But what would happen to Mother was less sure, her pneumonia could still go either way. We needed to think about what to do.

Nigel and Liz insisted that we should go. They knew how much it meant to us after the year and eight months we'd just gone through, and knowing that it would be restorative for us both. This was so generous of them.

No doubt for us all there was the unspoken thought that it might be our last holiday together. Although the ablation would extend my life, being denied systemic chemo suggested my future looked pretty limited.

> In the world, but not quite of it. Glitzy shops display new fashions, girls pass by in slinky summer styles. But my biggest treat is tea in a café, watching it all go by.

We followed up Dr Gillams' suggestion. Our GP would refer me to an oncologist at University College Hospital London. But if we went to Greece it would be hard to pursue the referral – and we'd learned that you really do keep having to push for things. Being a 'difficult patient' is at times the best option. Again, Liz stepped into the breach, offering to follow things up while we were away.

We were to fly to Kefalonia from Gatwick, staying with Nigel the night before. By great fortune – or was it more than that? – we would go close by the hospital Mother was in. As I was feeling so much better we would visit her. By now she was failing to respond to treatment, and it was looking likely that she would not survive.

Again, in consultation with Nigel and Liz, we decided to still go away. I had been with my father when he died, which I had always hoped to be. For some reason I felt all right about the possibility of not being there when Mother died, knowing my siblings were alongside her.

Whenever I tuned in to her, I sensed she had already detached to a large extent from her body. I saw her above the body, encased in light, and seemed to be shown that she was being held, cared for.

We visit her in hospital. A tiny, frail old lady lies in a bed on a ward. All tubes and drips have been removed. She is being given the care she needs for her body to let go of the being who is my mother in this life.

I hold her hand, speak to her. I can tell she knows me, even though she is apparently unconscious. She moves her head and arm towards me. I know this may be my last time with her, and seek to reassure her and remind her of good things in her life, times we have shared, and encourage her to be at peace.

> Sailboats catch the sun, tiny in the fine expanse of Plymouth Sound. Further out a naval ship's jagged outline is dark under thundery clouds. May those many beings who have ventured forth from here be at peace.

The next morning we wake in Kefalonia. Breakfast on the sunlit balcony, overlooking azure sea.

Nigel phones. Mother died this morning.

The morning Mother died I was in Greece, looking out from a small harbour to the island of Ithaca, that land known in legend as the home to which the traveller longs to return.

A beautiful white ship set out towards Ithaca,. moving so slowly I could hardly tell that it was departing. But it gradually grew smaller, moving around a headland, until I could barely see it. Closing my eyes in the warm sun, the ship had disappeared into Ithaca when I looked again. It had reached home.

Mother, now that you have left our shores may your journey be peaceful and may you be welcomed home.

Our two weeks in Kefalonia are clearly going to be very different from any previous holiday.

Chapter 23

Life and death had never seemed so closely linked before. We were in a stunningly lovely place, yet my mother had just died and I knew that I might soon too.

From our balcony we could see a small harbour, the sea and the mountains of Ithaca. I imagined Odysseus finally returning there after his long journeys, the white sails of his boat against the blue sky, just as I could see now.

There was a timelessness, yet I was acutely aware of how limited my own time might be. As Chetan said, it was time to open myself to greater mysteries. This would be not just a holiday, for fun and recuperation, but a kind of retreat too. I hoped that Chetan would be able to find the rest and relaxation he so badly needed.

I had brought Roshi Joan's *Being with Dying* book with me. This became of huge importance to me. Her words opened up my yearning to be more at ease with death. It may not sound like holiday reading, but was absolutely what I needed to know about. That we are always dying, that we are always letting go, that it just might be possible to move towards it with trust and expansiveness.

We fell into a routine of breakfast on the balcony, a little yoga and meditation, walking down to the harbour or to the stunning little beach nearby. I watched myself being full of joy one moment, then stabbed with pain at the memory of past holidays and the possibility of this being the last one, and then reminding myself to return to this moment.

Such a hard mixture of feelings to contain - the joy of being here, in this beautiful place, being with Chet and feeling so cherished by him, and today a huge amount of grief - that life is so brief, may soon end for me, Mother's death, the extreme delicacy of life, its fleetingness.

How can I be with this? I know the answer is about being here now, with what is, but 'what is' is also grief right now.

I let go of fear. I dwell in the present moment, giving thanks for this day, this moment, this moment.

The sun is coming through after a stormy night.

And Roshi Joan's words were giving me new tools, to help myself and to feel I may be helping others:

May loving kindness fill you and heal you.
May you and all beings be free from pain and sorrow.
May joy fill and sustain you.
May you accept things as they are.

We soaked up the warm spring sunshine, lazed along the harbour front looking through the clear water at the tiny fishes. There was good fresh food in the tavernas, though they were expensive so we cooked at home too. Chetan has always been a good cook, and to my delight loves cooking on holiday with the lovely local foods. I'd given up drinking wine, always a part of a holiday meal, but didn't feel the loss. There was too much else to enjoy, and I found I really enjoyed just seeing Chetan having a glass and relaxing.

Since chemo I couldn't stand very hot sun – my skin would burn easily – so late April sun in Greece was just perfect. I hardly needed to wear my tatty old sun hat that Chetan thought would look better on one of the Greek donkeys.

> I peel back my T-shirt so sunshine can nourish my abdomen. Still surprised by its new topography, my fingers trace long ridges, bumps, numb places. I'm proud of my body.

The island was studded with brilliantly coloured wild flowers, and the tallest geraniums I had ever seen. On May Day the village was bedecked with garlands, and young people performed athletic circle dances. We were delighted to just sit and people watch.

The holiday was like a retreat, but one filled with beautiful landscape, clear blue sea, sunshine, tavernas, reading, sinking into a very loving space with Chetan.

One morning though I woke feeling great sorrow in my heart. I sat on the balcony and did a meditation I had been reading about in *Being with Dying.* Tonglen meditation has been a great gift to me.

Breathing difficult feelings into my heart, so that a metal sheath around the heart cracks open, allowing the sorrow and grief to be absorbed, then breathing out lightness, fresh air, all the goodness from one's life. Doing that in relation to one's own suffering, then that of a beloved, someone you watch dying, then watching yourself dying. Very, very powerful. Felt like my heart - or the tight band of sorrow around it - was cracking open. Painful, but a relief too, to see some of the excruciating emotion from having this illness being absorbed into the vast space of the heart.

I seemed to be looking deeper and deeper into the depths of a wound - raw, deep, opening up like the centre of a flower, but very tender, painful, injured. Then breathing out, feeling the lightness, airiness, goodness that has been - and is - in my life. Letting that expand out of me, still painful and raw, but with a sense of wonder at how the breaking open of the heart through sorrow could allow the joy, the good, to flow forth.

I wondered if suffering breaks open something in us about an understanding of goodness, of love, of unity. The existence of suffering is so hard to accept and understand, but it does exist; and I was starting to see that, even in its presence, so too do joy and openness.

I painted the experience. It helped release a little more, though

I found working in the small sketchbook I'd brought much less freeing than the big boards I'd been using. And then to lunch, sitting in the sun with my beloved beside the blue sea.

Tonglen meditation has continued to be a powerful tool for me. Sometimes it is my own suffering that I breathe into my heart, before breathing life's goodness out from it. And sometimes I've felt able to breathe in other people's suffering, and send the joy from my heart and life to them.

At times I've found it really helpful as a way of not reacting in such a defensive or hostile way if Chetan and I are at odds with each other. When I've been able to catch myself, I've sometimes seen his pain beneath whatever would have tended to make me angry, and been able to breathe the pain into my heart, allow it to be there, then breathe life's goodness out to him. This isn't about controlling him or anyone. Far from it. It's about acknowledging the suffering that's within us all, and hoping to be with it, if not transform it. More than anything, it's been about seeing *my* own habitual responses of defensiveness and blame, and working towards finding more compassionate responses.

I spoke with Nigel and Liz on the phone. They were sorting out Mother's funeral. I did feel guilty about them having to do so much, but knew they were lovingly supporting me in doing this. Liz also mentioned that she was still trying to get me an appointment at UCH, but hadn't managed so far. I didn't hold out much hope of it being any time soon.

One morning I was put on the spot when Chetan said he thought I was wanting him to 'take this all away' from me. Was he right, did I think he could magically save me from my fate? I tried not to react by just denying it, and to see what the truth of it was.

To my surprise I found that, while it would be wonderful if he *could* take it all away (a cure would be great!), and that his being with me through this was a gift beyond words, I wouldn't want what I was going through to be taken from me. It *was* my process, I was learning so much through it. Though devastating at times, there were jewels in it which I treasured and would not give away for anything. That was quite a revelation.

> *In the passage from life to death… your old identity is thrashed like grain, and a new life may grow from the brokenness of your past and the breaking open of the present. Dying and being with dying are threshold experiences with the potential to destroy our self-clinging as they liberate us into a larger space.*
> *– Roshi Joan Halifax*

One night on Kefalonia I dreamt again of dying.

I was in a café with an old couple who were trying to sell all their possessions, including a car. They seemed very gentle and at ease.

Then I was walking along the side of a hill, on the edge of the snowline. My companion was anxious about getting to work, but I felt relieved that I no longer had to worry about it. I was heading towards the house of a healer friend, enjoying being the first to step in the fresh snow.

Then in the distance I heard voices singing a song that I really loved but hadn't heard for a long time. The singing was coming from a train, in which I could see the old couple. They looked very happy and relaxed.

This dream, which I knew was about death and dying, was much happier than previous ones. The old couple had let go of earthly things. They could no longer go anywhere else without their car, they had to get on the train, which seemed to be about travelling to a new life. In the dream my walking companion hadn't recognised the song, she was full of concern for everyday matters, but I had. I knew it was coming from people who were leaving their bodies, travelling on.

Although it was difficult, I felt pleased to have seen the old couple completely at ease with the journey away from this life. It was a natural thing for them. And if I was on an edge place myself – of the snow, the hillside, perhaps of life – at least I recognised the beauty and familiarity of the singing, which would one day call to me. Calling me back, perhaps, as it was already familiar.

> *One who is free of fear knows that at the deepest level of realisation there is no suffering, no birth, no death. Each moment is new and complete – right now being born, right now dying. All phenomena are in flux. Riding the waves of impermanence, the elements come together as form and dissolve into formlessness. In some sense we are never born; we will never die.*
> *– Roshi Joan Halifax*

I collect small, brilliant-white round pebbles from the beach. I need nine. The water is that pure, clear turquoise of the Greek islands. Still cold, so early in the year, but all I want to do is sit beside it, watch the goats climbing on the headland, look out towards Ithaca, be with Chetan.

I make a small circle with eight of the pebbles and place the ninth in the centre. It is my medicine wheel, set out to mark each of the eight main compass directions, and the centre of all things.

I sit in front of each direction, asking for guidance:

East: My guide Eagle Owl shows me where I am now. He gives me a lively young horse which I ride bareback, feeling free and alive in the wind. I ride fast, relishing the freshness, and when I'm complete I return to my tribe where they care for my weakness, hold and nourish me.

West: I am reminded to do vipassana breathing meditation. And sit upright, literally and metaphorically, for courage.

North: I need to 'get my house in order' – sort out paperwork, find a sense of completeness.

South: To allow the tears too, and more important, allow being cared for, knowing I am *always*, at all times, held in love like a beloved child.

South-east: Look again at Atisha's nine principles of death, which I had been reading about in *Being with Dying*. And eat good food; nourish the body.

North-west: Learn to trust – that I am part of an ancient path, and have been here (through death) many times before.

South-west: A reminder that there is no need to be in thrall to the medical world, that I had already faced the most difficult things there are. To know that *I* can choose, and to choose what feels *good*.

North-east: To let my goodness flow out to others, to give out.

Sitting in the circle, quietly waiting to see what came, I had a great sense of trust, of being guided. Some people see spirits and angels, and I do not doubt their experience. I don't see these, but I have often felt that guidance has been there with me. I have asked, and it has been given.

Our last day in Kefalonia. A beautiful day, though with difficult moments too. In the morning just being in the harbour, blue sky and sea, sitting watching the fishing boats, pastel-coloured buildings, eating Greek cake in our favourite taverna.

Knowing we will be leaving soon is a bit upsetting. But the time here has been about learning more about being in the moment with 'not knowing', feeling again the goodness in my life, having wonderful times and connections with Chet which have been unbelievably precious and away from everyday concerns.

And seeing the last eighteen months in a new perspective a bit - the scariness and awfulness of it. Letting that be in the past, so that I can be with what is right now.

So why have I been upset? Perhaps just an ending, reminding me of one day a permanent ending.

In the evening a walk to our little beach, sitting on the rocks as the sun went down, watching the clear water, goats on the rocks.

And then - even more wonders - back at the apartment watching a full moon rising above the mountains of Ithaca. At first in the pink twilight, then getting brighter and brighter as the darkness deepened. Reflection of the moon across the still sea - and then a ship outlined by its bright lights, sailing through the moon's pathway. Just to add to the joy and wonder, I heard wonderful birdsong - could it possibly have been a nightingale?

Enjoy it to the full, *be* in it each moment.

Chapter 24

I don't know how she's done it. Liz has managed to arrange a hospital appointment for me at UCH for two days after we get back from Kefalonia. She's brilliant.

It's also just a few days until Mother's funeral, so we stay with Nigel and Judi, rather than return to Devon straight away. It's a poignant time. I'm touched by all that Nigel, Judi and my niece Hannah do for us, and all that they and Liz have done to prepare for the funeral. We sit together in the sunny garden, going through the service, adding suggestions, getting upset with each other, mopping up the tears, even laughing.

> On the train, returning from hospital. Two tired children cry inconsolably. Minutes later they're laughing. I'm not very different.

It makes me think that I should soon put down some thoughts of what I would like for my funeral. Perhaps it is not far off. I'd like to make some suggestions – some poems, something I'll write myself, music I love, readings from Osho – but without taking away from what others want too.

But right now, a hospital appointment.

Although my referral was to UCH, I was to see a Dr Bridgewater, consultant oncologist, at North Middlesex Hospital with which it is affiliated. It didn't look promising. Sprawling and run-down, wires dangling along dishevelled dark corridors. But improvements were underway.

Another waiting room. All those anxious people again, including me and Chetan. Surely this scruffy place isn't going to come up with anything more than I was last offered at Plymouth – which was nothing, just palliative care to alleviate the worst symptoms as I slide towards death.

At last we're called in. Dr Bridgewater's support nurse is

warm and welcoming. I like her. But I still doubt they'll be able to help.

When Dr Bridgewater comes in I go through the now lengthy story of my illness. He probes, makes notes, listens carefully as I outline all that has happened. That I am now without hope of any further medical intervention.

'I can't see why you can't have second-line chemo, it hasn't been tried,' he says.

I am completely dumbfounded.

Am I being given yet another chance of life?

There's more. I can't quite believe that Dr Bridgewater is actually suggesting various options. First there's the second-line chemo: drugs of 'second choice' really, but which haven't been used before and therefore shouldn't present problems of resistance. It would be administered via a PICC line – an intravenous line from a box containing the chemo, strapped to the body. There was also a drug related to Avastin which had recently undergone trials and would soon be on the 'approved' list.

First, though, he wants me to have a PET scan. This will give a clearer image of what is going on than the CT or MRI scans.

We leave the hospital in a state of slightly delirious shock and joy. The prospect of chemo is far from pleasant, but it certainly helped before so I guess I will have it.

Before we set off from the hospital we have a drink in the cafeteria. I no longer care about the surroundings; I just give thanks to all the wonderful people working there.

Sannyas is a pilgrimage.
A pilgrimage from the dark night of the soul toward the dawn of the spirit.
It is not a ritual, it is an inner revolution.
It is not a formality, it is a love affair.

Unless it is something from your very heart it won't work.
It is not a question of believing.
It is not a question of intellectual conviction.
It is a question of falling in love, with something which one can feel but which one cannot understand by intellect itself.
It is a quantum leap.
– *Osho*

A couple of days later it was Mother's funeral. She had rarely spoken of her death, perhaps like most of us not believing she would die one day, but had once told me she would like to be buried in a woodland site. There was just such a place close to Bristol. It felt right, as did the whole of the occasion. Her body was in a wicker coffin interwoven with flowers, and as it was laid into the ground the sadness was balanced with a feeling of rightness, of her having lived a full life which had come to its natural end, and relief that she had not had to suffer any longer.

And so we returned home, after three weeks in which I had seen my mother dying, had a beautiful, loving and moving time with Chetan in Kefalonia, seen a new oncologist and been told I could have more treatment, and gone to Mother's funeral. No wonder it was so lovely to see the cats again, hold them tight.

A few days later I was back in London, for the PET scan. This felt like real high-tech stuff. Before it I had to drink a solution then lie absolutely still for almost an hour. Another good opportunity to practise meditation! The scan seemed to go on for ages.

And now today, sitting in bed with Chet, with Fred the ginger cat on the bed. Yesterday's scan was a bit scary, not just the procedure but wondering what they'll find.

Try to stay with the present moment, anchoring with the breath. And remembering too Atisha's precepts about the impermanence of life, the not knowing. Thank you for this moment.

A few days later I was having my usual after-lunch snooze, during which I would listen to a visualisation or a healing. Chetan was always keen to not disturb me during this, so when he came in with the phone I knew it was important. It was the lovely support nurse phoning me about the PET scan. There were 'hot spots' on the colon and liver, she said, but not in the lymph or anywhere else.

That was great news. There was more. They wanted to *operate on my colon*. This would be followed up later with more RFA on the liver.

I didn't sleep much after that!

After all the hoping that one day I would have an operation on the colon. From the very start I had hoped for that, only to be told repeatedly that it was not an option because of the state of my liver, which was far more imminently life-threatening. Professor Vogl had suggested it as a possibility once the liver had been treated, only for that hope to be dashed once new tumours appeared on the liver. I had long since put such a hope out of my thoughts, and now here it was, being offered.

I could only give thanks from the depths of my heart. I didn't really doubt that an operation was a good thing, that surely the removal of the primary tumour must help. I thanked the medical people, all my beloved ones who had helped me get to this point, and the guidance from who knew where that had brought me here.

Will it really extend my life considerably?

There were fears and worries of course, as it is a major operation. I wondered if it would be very painful, how long it would take to recover from, whether it might even spread the cancer through disrupting the body so greatly. But I would be able to discuss all this with Dr Bridgewater when I went to see him in a few days. The operation was likely to be soon – within the next couple of weeks or so.

I need to start talking to my body about the operation, accepting and welcoming it. Hard to even imagine my body being opened up and part of me - a very fundamental part! - being removed. But it did happen before, when I had my appendix removed, and that actually saved my life.

I've lost a bit of the calm I found in Kefalonia. Not surprising with so much happening. So try to tune back into the breath, the watchful place.

Two weeks after Mother's funeral I dreamt of her. She was working in a café, which I was surprised she could do. But she was being supported by a lovely warm, solid woman, and others. She was still a bit withdrawn and confused, but less than she had been following the stroke. Her hair was dark again. I knew she was receiving great care, and gradually getting better.

I wondered if this was indeed what was happening to her.

The next night's dream was more painful. Walking along a sunny road I heard someone shouting my name. It was Liz, shouting 'Di, Di, Di' – which is what she calls me – and absolutely distraught. It was so painful, and I knew I couldn't carry on along the road just then, but had to turn back to be with her.

Is this connected with the op? That I'm turning back from dying - from walking away from her? If so, I give thanks. Maybe I can still love and support Liz more in this life, in whatever way is possible.

Perhaps something deep within me *was* choosing to live, and I was being given every blessed opportunity to do so.

Chapter 25

If I thought things had taken a new and better turn, I was in for more surprises.

When Chetan and I saw Dr Bridgewater to discuss the operation and ablation, he said that if I had those done there was a chance I could be *cancer-free*. I could hardly take this in, yet he of all people would never say such a thing if it wasn't a possibility.

The treatment in Germany had been very effective, Dr Bridgewater said. The PET scan showed that the tumours Professor Vogl had treated were now calcified – non-active.

It was lovely to have this affirmation of what had always felt like the right thing, but had been so dismissed within the NHS.

The operation would be in just two or three weeks, the ablation to the liver a month after that.

We reeled out of the hospital, ecstatic at this news, not quite knowing what it meant, fearful about the operation, but mostly just joyful. We fell into the nearby British Museum, bathing in its glorious treasures and especially the Buddhas, reminding me of stillness and impermanence amidst this unexpected hope for more life.

Do I *dare* to hope? I can hardly take in this turnaround, from being told just a few weeks ago there was nothing left but palliative care, and now to be told this. I think my mind can hardly cope with it. Which is also a pretty good message - it's now time in my life to really work with *not* being in the mind all the time (which I am), to learn to just be. To be in the present, the now, with the breath, in the now, now, now.

I open myself to new possibilities through this op.

Just three days later Lisa was visiting me to give me a craniosacral session. The phone rang. It was UCH. The operation would be in a week's time, sooner than I'd expected. We'd been planning a few days away before it, but when the hospital offered me a later date I knew I didn't want to delay it.

Suddenly it seemed horribly real. I cried. Mostly from fear, but relief too. The cranio session was perfect timing, as was Lisa's calming presence.

The op also meant that I would miss a workshop I'd been planning to attend. It was about phowa, a Buddhist practice for approaching death. I had read about it in Roshi Joan Halifax's book. I wanted to have a practice that would take me into a peaceful death – and beyond, and phowa seemed to offer that. But now it would have to wait a while.

> On a so-beautiful-it's-almost-corny June morning I sing as I walk through the garden. Halfway across the lawn, to the bench where I will meditate, my heart skips a beat. I gasp. What if the liver tumour grows through a blood vessel? Joy and anguish, I sit and watch them both.

Two days later we were back at UCH again, for meetings and tests prior to the op. I met the surgeon, who was kind and reassuring. He told me there was a chance I would have to have a stoma bag fitted, but he hoped it would be possible to fully rejoin the bowel where a section had been removed. This would not be known until the operation. It should be possible to do the operation as a keyhole procedure, meaning it would all heal much more quickly.

What I hadn't expected was another incredible bit of news. I was told that there was now a plan to *operate on my liver*. This was almost more than I could take in. How was this possible after all I'd been told before – that there was too much tumour in the liver for this to ever be a possibility? In those horribly memorable words of a doctor in Exeter, 'No surgeon in the world would ever operate on your liver.' How could he have been so wrong? But such questions were for another day.

An operation on the liver!! It's just extraordinary. I feel I am being showered on, with gifts of life, and that there is *more life for me.*

I am so, so grateful. I know all sorts of things can happen, and of course it can come back, but what a gift right now. Scary too of course, although all the meetings at UCH were very reassuring.

Right now, I'm just grateful.

The liver op would probably be six to eight weeks after the colon one, which seemed pretty daunting. They would remove the left lobe of the liver, and some of the right lobe, leaving about 50 per cent of it. Apparently you can manage with just a third of your liver. Scary but wonderful.

I felt in awe of all these people, many of whom I would never meet, who had dedicated themselves to their work, their learning, which was giving me this opportunity.

Before this hospital visit I had decided to write a round-robin letter to all my friends and family, telling them about the colon op. I hoped they wouldn't mind such a letter, as I really needed to thank them for all the support they'd given me so far, which had got me to this point – and now to ask for more. Now I had to change the letter, to say that this first operation would be followed by an even more major one. I could still hardly believe it.

Now, though, it was just a few days until the colon op. I looked at my body in the mirror. It would soon be marked and scarred, never the same again. But that was fine, how could I complain about such trivia? I said goodbye to how it looked now. What was a bit less fine was the thought that very soon I would probably be in pain.

Right now I need to put aside thinking about the liver op and put all my energy into this colon one. Being positive, looking forward to healing, bringing light into my body, *knowing all is well.*

The day before we travelled up to London for the op I packed to the sound of Mozart's *Magic Flute.* Any operation has its risk of mortality, however small, and the extraordinary sounds of Mozart's divine music reminded me of the wonders of life.

Early morning. We walk to the hospital from our nearby hotel. I try to watch my breath, feel my feet on the pavement. In time with my breath I mentally recite Joan Halifax's words:

Breathing in, I calm body and mind.
Breathing out, I let go.
Dwelling in the present moment
This is the only moment.

Or I use Thich Nhat Hanh's words:

In, out.
Deep, slow.
Calm, ease.
Smile, release.
Present moment, only moment.

These reminders will become my refuge during my stay in hospital.

More paperwork, then a meeting with the stoma nurse. He shows me what the entry point for a stoma bag will look like, if that's needed. I'm quite shocked, it looks so ugly. I very much hope I won't need one, though also commit to accepting it with positivity if it proves necessary.

Then at last my name is called. I say goodbye to Chetan, and go off with the theatre nurse. He's the perfect person for this job, leading me into the unknown with some good-humoured banter. I put on the hospital gown, leave my clothes behind and walk almost as naked as the day I was born towards the operating room. I feel small and vulnerable as I walk down the corridor. I call on all the love that has been sent to me so many times, wrap it around me like a cocoon of light, and know that I am always safe. I am walking towards the operating theatre escorted by a whole throng of friends known and unknown.

Chapter 26

I'm crying in the chapel. It's the fifth day since the colon op, and I've already managed to get to the ground floor of the hospital, where the little chapel is. To get there I've walked – very warily – through the bustle of people, happy to be stepping back into life. How wonderful that the hospital has provided this sacred place, a chapel where I can allow tears which seem to be a mixture of gratitude and shock. And I do give thanks.

I hadn't had to have a stoma. I hazily remember being told this good news as I came round from the op. About ten inches of colon had been removed and rejoined, all with keyhole surgery. What a marvel.

The pain was really well controlled, with an epidural which was removed after a few days. Pain management was clearly given high priority – in the middle of one night when I did have pain two specialist pain medics arrived to help me, and adjusted the epidural.

I can't quite believe that the primary cancer is no longer in my colon. I'm pretty scared about the next op, but I know that right now I just need to be putting everything into recovering from this.

My mantras for being in the present moment – which somehow *was* always bearable – were my staunch allies.

I was overwhelmed and humbled by all the love and support I received. Flowers and cards arrived from friends; many visitors came including sannyasin friends I hadn't seen since living in London years before. The connections run deep. My relatives cradled me with their supportive network; I was strengthened by them all. Each person's gesture brought me a step further back into life.

> Desolate and grieving, I cry for help to the Buddhas. A butterfly lands right over my heart. The tabby cat settles on my lap.

When I had started chemo I had avoided much involvement with the other patients, sensing the need to work with my own thoughts, feelings and healing, deal with my own shock. That had gradually changed and now, in the hospital, relating with other patients was precious.

I was in a little side-ward with three other women. Though we were all very ill, there was an undercurrent of compassion between us. The elderly lady who spoke no English made sure her relatives shared homemade sweetmeats with us all. My neighbour who had hardly any intestine left was warm and kind, and the lady struggling with thoughts of suicide as well as a serious medical condition told me of her love of God, and asked her priest to come to my bedside and pray with me, which he did.

When I was weepy, a nurse stroked my hand. When I felt scared and alone I looked at my cards and flowers, remembered that day's visitors, and knew I was loved. When I needed to still myself I tuned in to my breath, to my inner being. I asked for help from Osho, using his name as a mantra. When I pined to be out of hospital I looked out of the ninth-floor window at the sights of London.

I tried to treat the time in hospital as an opportunity to be present, in the moment, whenever I could. And when it was possible that always helped, especially with fear.

There is a vastness beyond the farthest reaches of the mind.
That vastness is my home.
That vastness is myself.
And that vastness is also love.
– Nisargadatta Maharaj

I was visited by Mr Imber, the surgeon who would operate on my liver. He told me that someone with my condition might expect to live about two years with 'conventional' treatments, but that with liver surgery life expectancy was more like five years. Only five, I thought! Ungrateful woman. I found it extraordinary that I was being offered this treatment, in this very down to earth, matter of fact way. I knew how lucky I was.

But I didn't dare think too much about more surgery. I had more pressing preoccupations, such as hoping I'd soon be able to go to the loo! I wouldn't be discharged until I had, so that it was clear the bowel was working. I could hardly believe that my 'new' bowel would know what to do. But one day, it did. I was so thankful I wanted to tell the world, but it was probably more information than the world wanted.

By the end of a week or so, I longed to go home. I had to have a CT scan done first, and unfortunately my vein ruptured when dye was injected into it, making my arm swell up like a marrow and causing much alarm to the medics. But by the next day it was clear that there were no serious side effects, and I was on my way home.

Wonderful to be out of the hospital. As the ambulance (which brought me all the way home!) drove along the motorway I caught a smell of new-mown grass, a real treat after being in the air-conditioned intensity of the hospital.

I may have been glad to get home, but I could tell that Chetan was under a lot of stress. Perhaps the operation had been a catalyst for it to surface. He had thought I might go to Nigel's for a few days after the op, and I hadn't quite taken it in that he really could have done with more time to himself. He was exhausted, and now I was home and full of needs.

The day after I got home my reading for the day from *Daily Word* said:

In this very moment, I claim my health and wholeness. Whether for a few minutes or life-changing moments, I take time to focus on and discern what is best for me. Such times for regeneration support the health of every cell and function of my body. During meditative prayer, concerns dissipate, answers come, and healing flows.

And as if that wasn't encouragement enough, the next day when I was starting to feel anxious about the liver op, the reading was:

As a creation of a loving Creator, I welcome new beginnings, which are new chapters in my own story of life. My faith in God's ever-present guidance is constant. And I go forward confident in my insights, my choices, and my actions… Goodness abounds, and I celebrate my freedom to begin anew.

It gave me a sense of confidence. I was making the right choice, and that choice would give me the freedom to 'begin anew' – or at least have yet another chance of longer life.

I was surprised to feel some grief for the part of my colon that had been removed. Though I was delighted to no longer have the primary, I also needed to give thanks to the part that had gone, and which had served me so well for most of my life.

The scarring was minimal, thanks to the keyhole surgery. And although there was still some pain, and I was weak and tired, the good food and air, and being back with Chetan, soon started to pick me up and to heal the shock to the body.

Live now.
Heal.
Know I am surrounded in love and light.

A few days after getting home it was midsummer solstice. I remembered being in Cornwall for solstice two years ago, when I had no idea of what was about to hit me. Or perhaps I did. That seemed almost like another life, so much had happened since then.

Then I thought of just the last three months, hardly able to believe what has happened in that time - being told by Professor Vogl there were new tumours, then Dr Daniel saying no more treatment, then Rosy Daniel suggesting Dr Gillams and the ablation with her, the referral to Dr Bridgewater, talk of chemo, the scan, the offer of operations - and the op I've now had. And of course Mother dying in the middle of this. No wonder I feel a bit wobbly! Thank goodness we had that wonderful two weeks in Kefalonia, it gave me such joy and a reserve to draw on. Thank you, thank you.

As well as the loss of a physical part of me, there was sometimes a sense of disempowerment. Just small things, like not being able to lift anything heavy, pull open a drawer, having to ask for help so much. These things would pass, but they were reminders of how much had changed. I was no longer that strong, independent person I thought myself to be. And now I needed to balance the 'doing' with resting, without feeling frustrated, or that I was a burden, or had to prove anything. Accepting what is, that I can no longer do what I took for granted, has proved to be ongoing work.

The last few days have been wonderful days of summer - lots of sitting in the garden, quite magical with the bees buzzing in and out of the flowers, the warmth, the dappled shade of the trees, the veg growing in the back garden.

I'd become so engrossed in my own stuff that I hadn't truly seen what had been happening with Chetan. In the few days since I'd come home we had been sparring a lot, just not really hearing each other. Or maybe I just wasn't hearing him, through the miasma of my preoccupation with my pain, my fear, my feeling sorry for myself.

I suddenly got it. I needed to listen to him, to see him and all that he had been carrying. He was exhausted physically, emotionally, mentally. I felt ashamed, knowing that he had given his life over to me in these two years and that all he had done for me was beyond thanks. I had taken his ability to cope with it all for granted. I knew I must be much more aware of his needs, for him to have time for himself when he wasn't having to pick up the pieces of my emotions, cook for me, do all those other many things – for him to live his life.

May Chetan be held in love.
May we live in peace and joy.

That night I dreamt of Chetan. I was just holding him, kissing him, feeling so much love for him. When I woke I prayed that I could be one bit as loving to him as he had been to me.

As fear arose about the next op, I asked for a visualisation to help me. My mind came up with what seemed like a corny image – a dark tunnel, with the faintest glimmer of light at the end of it. But it worked. There *was* light there, shining on trees and grass. And then I saw that the walls of the tunnel were not as dark as they first appeared. They were lined with flowers, friends, good things. I was being told that even in the darkness I was being supported.

My birthday. I've made it to fifty-seven! There were times when I doubted I would, and of course that has always been possible. Thank you God.

I give thanks to all my beloveds, Chet, my family, my friends, the medical people who got me here. And that does include *all* of them!

Jo and Fran are coming for lunch today. It's a lovely day of sunshine and showers. I give thanks for my life. I gather the fullness of it to me, like a rich wine of all I have known, experienced, learnt, lived. I have been, and am, incredibly fortunate in this life.

During the day I watched my mind making difficulties: 'How many more birthdays?', 'This is more than I can bear', fear about what lay ahead. But I was utterly spoilt, and bathed in generosity.

Now
That
All your worry
Has proved such an
Unlucrative
Business,
Why
Not
Find a better
Job.
– Hafiz

I have heard the date of the liver operation. It's in just ten days' time, much sooner than I'd expected. It suddenly feels real. Oh God, what if I get swine flu, what if, what if… I encourage my body to welcome the op, and to be open to this experience as part of my life.

Janet, my healer friend from BCHC, sends me a CD to prepare for an operation. It's a visualisation of everything going well, connecting with and trusting the medical staff, seeing the positive outcome and healing. It really does help.

A week before the op Chetan gives me seven parcels wrapped in shimmering pink paper, one for each day. What a lovely thing to do. Each one contains a little treat – a bar of chocolate, soap, and in one there's a book. It's *Grace and Grit* by Ken Wilber, a renowned writer on metaphysical matters, and tells the story of his wife's cancer from which she eventually died. I know there will be much learning in it.

I meet Mr Imber a few days before the op. There's excitement, disbelief, as well as the fear. I'm really thrown though when I hear that a biopsy after the first op has shown cancer still in the nodes. I'll need chemo after the liver op to 'mop it up'.

It's upsetting. I have to change my mindset yet again, having thought I'd be on a steady road to recovery after this. Sometimes it all feels too much. But then it changes again. A friend rings, and reminds me of what I have in my life.

I pray that through this operation my life may blossom with new life.

Remember to be the witness.

With two days to go before the operation I sleep badly. Chetan helps me look at all the fears – the hospital, needles, being opened up, that I might die, pain, chemo. He encourages me to witness them, talks me through it. We spend a day by the sea, letting it all blow away a bit. Then there is a wonderful lunch with sannyasin friends. Their love and the depth of meditation around them really changes how I'm feeling. Atosh gives me a lovely tiny crystal angel to take with me, and Jitindriya insists I take her gorgeous pashmina. I know it's a favourite of hers, and she is giving it to me to wrap me in love. It's become my favourite ever since.

It's the day before the op. Though aware of dread, I feel fairly calm and centred. If I die, may I be prepared and at peace. If I live, may I be in joy and gratitude, and live each moment. My beloved Chet is dozing in bed. He is so beautiful. Thank you for our lovely trip to the sea yesterday, and for so much you have given me.

And so we go into this next bit of adventure.

Chapter 27

Waiting. It's agonising. We've arrived at the hospital in good time. I've walked in feeling quite good, warrior-like, trying to be in the moment. But now I'm told there's a chance there won't be a bed for me because of the swine flu epidemic. If there isn't, the operation won't happen.

After what seems like hours I'm told it is happening. The same cheerful nurse who took me to the operating theatre before takes me there now. I change into my robe, feeling again like a tiny dot, asking that Osho, my spirit helpers, the love from everyone, surround me as I walk a bit shakily towards the operating room.

This will be a big operation, several hours. It's not possible to do it by keyhole surgery, so there will be large incisions. One-half of my liver will be removed, a wedge taken out of the other half, possibly the gall bladder removed too, according to how it looks. I'm having a 'left lateral hepatectomy, and a wedge resection on the right side'. Bleeding is a major factor in a liver op. But I know this is a highly skilled team.

Here's Chetan. He's shaved, looks different. And I seem to have been pushed through a solid wall on my bed. Slowly I realise the operation is over, I'm in intensive care. The procedure was over six hours long.

The next day I was told I had MRSA. This was a bit of a blow, but I was so drugged up it didn't affect me too much. Because of this I would have to be put in a room by myself, in isolation. I was sad about this at first, not to be in contact with others, but then decided I must regard it as a retreat. While I waited for a room to become available I spent an extra night in intensive care, surrounded by sounds of people in distress, but feeling very secure in the care of the staff.

As I became more with it, I learnt that the whole of the left lobe had indeed been removed, along with a wedge from the right lobe. They hadn't needed to remove the gall bladder, but weren't able to take away every bit of tumour, as that would have left me with too little liver.

I had a pretty big L-shaped incision down and across my abdomen, held together by an alarming-looking row of large steel staples. An epidural was again doing a great job with the pain.

My 'retreat room' was like a penthouse suite, with fantastic views across London to St Paul's, the London Eye. I could watch the vast sky during the day, and the lights of London when I was awake in the night.

I had lots of wonderful visitors again, boosting and encouraging me, bringing the outside world in to uplift me. Even so, after a few days it did start feeling a bit like *Groundhog Day* in my little retreat. My iPod was a real resource – I could listen to meditations, visualisations, healing chants.

I asked to be visited by the chaplain. Even though I'm not a Christian I wanted that contact with spirituality, the chance to pray. I hope I wasn't abusing the good man. I was reminded of my childhood upbringing as a Christian, and was glad for having had that basis of spirituality in my early life.

For two or three nights in a row I had a strange sensation, always at about the same time, of someone else being in the room, even though I knew there wasn't anyone else there. I was sure I could hear and feel someone right next to me, rustling the bedclothes. Was it the drugs making me hallucinate, or was I more sensitive than usual. I'm not sure. But by the fourth night, when it happened again, I'd convinced myself it was one or more beings who had died in the hospital, and for some reason had not been able to allow their soul to leave. I prayed that they might be taken to the light. It didn't happen again.

Having the single room turned out to be a blessing. It was peaceful, far more recuperative than being on a busy ward. Plus the fantastic view. I was treated with body washes and antibiotics for the MRSA. I must have only just contracted it, as it was only present in my nose. I was lucky; it did go quickly.

So now I'm in bed for the evening, later to fall into the arms of the Buddha as I sleep. With gratitude and just daring to hope a bit more. Dare I?!

Amazingly, I was only in hospital for a week and a day. I was discharged once I was able to totter cautiously, with encouragement from a physio, up and down a couple of steps.

Back home. Time to *really* start healing.

Walking (very slowly!) up the path, back from hospital, seeing the loveliness of the garden, knowing that any minute I would see Chet again, it flashed through my thoughts that of course I had known there was always a possibility I wouldn't make it back again. And then here I was, having gone through this immense thing. Yes, I did go through that dark tunnel, and yes, I was surrounded by love, support on so many levels. That makes me weep now.

The first night home I woke up screaming, shouting 'Mum' out loud, from a nightmare about an intruder in the house who might attack us. A pretty good analogy for what had just happened to my body. And the pain and discomfort were reminders for quite a while.

My GP came to see me the day after I came home. She sat and held my hand for ages. How many doctors would do that?

Carrie came that day too, and gave me a kinesiology session while I was in bed. It really helped; I felt much calmer, less jangled and peculiar afterwards.

My appetite was minute. The tiniest amount left me feeling as though I'd eaten a ten-course meal. I learnt later that the liver grows back to its full size – though not necessarily the same shape – within a couple of weeks. Extraordinary. So maybe that had something to do with my appetite. As it returned I had a craving for eggs and cheese; my body must have been needing protein. One time I could only manage half a small, cooked beetroot, but Chetan presented it as though it was Cordon Bleu cooking.

To help cope with the pain and shock I kept a note of any new thing I managed to do each day. I thought it would be helpful in low moments to be able to see that I *was* a little better every day. In the first few days there was managing to get up and down stairs twice in a day. I progressed to walking as far as the cattle grid, then to the telegraph pole on the green. My first trip out was to Ali's to see her gorgeous new kittens, full of life. Less than three weeks after the op, I was having a very gentle walk on the beach.

It was a joy to lie in the warm sand, listening to the waves, feeling the breeze. It blew away some of the awfulness I still felt, replacing it with the hope of moving more and more into the joy of life.

Watching Chetan walking along the water's edge, I felt a sadness, wondering if this is how it will be one day - just him - and praying that whatever happens he will be cared for, be happy, be ok.

Jean visits. We walk very slowly by the river, eating ice cream, me learning more from her about Tibetan Buddhism. I ask her if she will be with me when I am dying. She says she will.

At the time it felt as though my recovery was taking ages, but looking back at my little diary it seems miraculous how fast it was.

Sept 8: (about 7 weeks after the op) 7.30 am - chi kung beside the river!
Sept 14: drove the car two miles.

Yet there was rage too. While my mind felt full of gratitude, something deep in me was ranting, furious. The catalyst for this was that we had planned to be in Cornwall with Liz for a few days, in what turned out to be the second week after the op. I was far too weak to go; and while my mind totally understood why, another part of me raged at being ill, weak, helpless, in pain, feeling like shit, vulnerable. Perhaps I should have been ashamed, having been given this wonderful chance, but I felt it needed to be acknowledged, released, as part of the healing process.

I drew a strange picture of a 'raging woman' rising up out of the hospital building, towering over it like a primeval goddess:

She's surrounded by all the new technology to help with the healing, but abhors it too, says it should never have come to this, to need all these aids to healing. Meanwhile, even through her rage, from within the hospital she is picking up, holding, healing and nurturing her beloved children.

I guess I was asking for her help.

Sitting in the garden, not denying those furious feelings are still there, but also enjoying the plants, sitting here, and the *knowledge* that I am much more than my body.

Help must have been there all the time. In a healing session with Helen I 'saw' a mesh or net of blue and gold light being put within my abdomen, holding it and re-establishing its structure as it should be. Then this peaceful state was replaced by rage at my condition, rising up as a huge energy through the earth, into my feet, right up through my body. Incredibly powerful.

I was being given a lesson. It was about taking responsibility for this energy, using it for the good, not dissipating it in blame and negativity.

There is yet another way that the imagination heals, and that is to enter into a moment of sensing the ecstatic truth of being absolutely and totally inseparable from every other aspect of creation. That moment itself is both the definition and purpose of healing. Sometimes physical problems disappear, and sometimes the patient dies. Either way, with the instant of connection, of unity, healing occurs.

– 'The Wounded Healer': Jeanne Achterberg

At the end of the session both Helen and I had a great sense of something very powerful, from another realm, still happening. I seemed to hear: 'To those who have been given so much, much may be asked.'

Chapter 28

Chetan and I are down by the river, chucking cones and twigs into it, watching them being swept away. It's two years today since I was diagnosed with cancer.

Our 'throwing it all away' ceremony is to let go of the pain and grief of that time. Then we set our intention for health, light and love, for a new part of the journey to begin. It's moving and powerful.

Let new health, new life and joy come to us.

And new things were happening, as I healed. Just four weeks after the op we were able to go to Cornwall in our little caravan, the first time we'd managed it all year. It meant a lot of work for Chetan because I was still so creaky, but it took us back into some kind of normality and enjoyment. The first night there we dined on delicious food, left over from a lunch that my old friend Diana had brought us. An edible reminder of all the support we'd been receiving.

It was painful too, being on holiday. I could only walk very short distances, would get tired and weepy. But we were there, in the sun.

I guess there's that undercurrent of how different everything is in my life now, the knowledge of death and wondering how long I may live, the absolute grief about that. I don't want to die, I can only pray that when that time does come I do feel acceptance and trust.

Perhaps that was connected with another dream I had of Chetan being seduced by a beautiful woman, full of youthful energy. In the dream I felt huge anger, and told her I would just kill her if she seduced him. I felt powerless. I also noticed she had a very slim waist, no doubt in contrast to my wound-bloated one!

Although I have never wanted to speculate about what Chetan might do after my death, these thoughts must have been there.

Coping with hospital appointments has been an ongoing torture. It has got easier, as I've become more used to the fear they engender, and have worked on relaxing, trying to be in the moment, breathe… When we got back from Cornwall I was due to go to London to see Dr Bridgewater and Mr Imber. I was fearful that I would hear that not all the tumour had been removed.

My fears proved correct. Mr Imber explained that there was more tumour present than had shown up on the PET scan, but he had not been able to remove any more of the liver as it would not have left me with enough. The extraordinary thing, though, was that because the liver regenerates it could be operated on again, and more removed. The thought of that was completely awful, but extraordinary too.

Apart from this news, seeing Mr Imber was an odd experience, lovely man though he is. Here was someone who had seen right inside me! It felt strangely intimate, that he had seen what was inside me when I hadn't myself.

Dr Bridgewater, whom I saw next, was much more upbeat. He said it was 'extremely positive' that they had managed to remove the primary tumour, and most of the active tumours in the liver.

I had also been dreading hearing about starting chemo, which I had been told would happen. But Dr Bridgewater said that although active cancer had been found in one of the calcified tumours (those treated by laser in Germany), the deposits of cancer which remained throughout the liver were inactive at present. So *I did not need chemo now.*

I was delighted. The dread of having to return to the awfulness of chemo, as soon as I'd got over the operations, had hung over me.

I would probably need chemo again at some time, Dr

Bridgewater said. He stressed that there were plenty of options if the cancer spread, such as a new drug that had been recently approved by NICE. There would be another scan in October. I immediately saw myself starting to worry about it, and brought myself back to healing now, getting better, releasing the final bits of cancer from my body. Letting them being washed away, as in our river ceremony.

How not to drop into feeling heartbroken, wanting to live? Holding it all - the preciousness of life and all I love in it, not wanting it to leak out, to disappear. I know the answer is being in the present, the now, but it's hard. It's hard.

We wandered out of the hospital into the hot late-August sun. I was exhausted. We sat on a bench in Fitzroy Square, and I laid my head on Chetan's lap. I rested in the comfort and love of him. The square was full of sunshine, people enjoying themselves, but I was also aware of 'ghosts'. We were sitting by Virginia Woolf's house, and there were reminders of many other famous and not-so famous people who had lived there. And me, I was just a little spark passing by at that moment.

I felt strangely numb. Maybe not quite daring to take in the good things, latching on to 'it could all come back again'. So now I need to change my mindset:

> *The primary cancer has gone. All the big liver tumours have gone. Yes, there's cancer in the liver and lymph but it is inactive.*

Keep it that way. Now is the time to move back into life, to let go of all this, to *live* again. Yes, I want to do that. To live joyfully, peacefully.

And now here at Liz's for a few days. Really lovely to be with them all. Time to rejoice.

Liz and I decided to make plans to have a little break together in the autumn. Perhaps a pampering weekend, maybe something more meditation based. We looked up all sorts of places. One of them was somewhere called Dzogchen Beara, a Tibetan Buddhist retreat centre in Ireland run under the auspices of the Tibetan teacher Sogyal Rinpoche, author of *The Tibetan Book of Living and Dying*. I saw that it ran a course called Living up to Dying. The description of the course instantly rang bells:

> *If we can only learn how to face death, then we'll have learned the most important lesson of life: how to face ourselves and so come to terms with ourselves, in the deepest possible sense, as human beings.*
> *– Sogyal Rinpoche*

It went on to say:

> *Contemplation of death is the cornerstone of all spiritual traditions. It helps us to sort out our priorities and to see what is truly meaningful for us. When we have the courage to face the fragility of life, we are rewarded with a far deeper appreciation of life's richness and beauty.*
>
> *In countless lectures and seminars around the world Sogyal Rinpoche has addressed the most important questions of living and dying, showing how what we call 'life' and what we call 'death' are parts of one single process... Through training in methods of meditation and contemplation we can step beyond superstitions and begin to approach death without fear, glimpsing what it is in us that survives death and is changeless. We can uncover a depth of peace, joy and confidence that transforms both life and death.*

The words went straight to my heart. I knew I wanted to go. And perhaps this would be a chance to learn phowa. The course was early November, more than two months away. I was determined to be strong enough by then to cope with the travel and the workshop.

I felt stronger every day while I was at Liz's. I was walking faster, managing a bit of chi kung and yoga. In my weepy moments Liz was there; we shared the pain of what was happening. She said she had envisioned me going 'to the edge of the precipice', having to look down into whatever was below, but not going over it.

One day I suddenly realised I was feeling at a bit of a loose end. My energy must be returning! I looked at what I wanted to do with my time, now that I was clearly starting to feel much better. I hoped I might be able to go back to the print workshop in autumn. And maybe start to do some writing. But what about? Certainly about the cancer, but would anyone want to read that? Maybe I would just do it for myself, maybe start it and see where it went.

On the train, going home from Liz's. Feel so much better than when I came a week ago. It has been a precious time with her - she's looked after me so beautifully, we've had lots of sharing times, often with plenty of tears.

Life seems so wonderful as I look out of the train at the beautiful late-summer landscape - the deep greens, the gold of the hay meadows, blue sky with some dark clouds. And feeling well.

Suddenly it feels as though all truly is well. That even when I die, all will be well, even the process of dying. But that is all future. Right now, enjoying this journey, the beauty of the land, feeling so loved by Liz and family, my friends - and looking forward to seeing Chet. It's quite strange that at the times I feel at my best - relaxed, easy - I also feel it easiest to contemplate death. As though right now is so fine that how could it be otherwise?

I wanted to get in touch with the part of me that truly knows how to heal. I told myself to open to the healing love of the divine; the operation had left me with a feeling of disconnection. I needed to come back to my body, my life. One day I found myself just screaming and screaming. I let myself carry on doing it, knowing it was coming from the depth of my body, releasing the feeling of being invaded – which it had been. Thank goodness we live in a remote place!

This quest to 'get back in touch with the divine' was answered in a healing session with Helen. During it I 'heard' the words, 'The divine is all around.' I knew this had come in response to my wish to feel connected. It was telling me that the connection had never gone. When I opened my eyes a beautiful light was playing on the ceiling, shaped just like an angel. I absolutely knew, at least for a moment, that the divine is truly in everything, even 'man-made' things. How could it be otherwise, when all comes from that source?

I started going again to chan – Chinese Buddhist meditation. When I first went, a few months before, I had at last found it possible to sit for an hour and a half, while the fear sometimes arose, and sometimes went again. It had given me a way to start being more at ease with just what is.

One night I dreamt that Pete, the meditation leader, gave me a great shove. I was a bit upset and really startled. I wondered what this was about, as Pete is the gentlest of men.

Dropping into my mind, my self, seeing where it takes me. Dropping down into the essence.

The message of the dream was about exploring meditation in a way I hadn't seen before. I was starting to see that meditation could be a light, joyful thing, an exploration of being. It was time to let the mind feel it was safe, by becoming used to what was there through meditation. And Pete had given me that metaphorical shove.

> *Sustained conscious attention severs the link between the pain-body and your thought processes and brings about the process of trans-*

mutation. It is as if the pain becomes fuel for the flame of your consciousness, which then burns more brightly as a result... the transmutation of the base metal into gold, of suffering into consciousness. The split within is healed, and you become whole again...

Stay present, and continue to be the observer of what is happening inside you. Become aware not only of the emotional pain but also of 'the one who observes', the silent watcher. This is the power of the Now, the power of your own conscious presence.
– Eckhart Tolle

On the anniversary of the attack on the Twin Towers in New York we watched a programme showing the madness, the consequences of hating to the point of insanity. But I knew it was no good pontificating, that I had responsibility too, to start with myself, cleanse myself, to be still, watchful and conscious, loving and accepting.

Next morning there was great news about Chetan. He had had a prostate biopsy, and it was clear. Great joy. We watched the swallows gathering on the wire, soon to fly off. Another extraordinary, miraculous event.

I
Do not
Want to step so quickly
Over a beautiful line on God's palm
As I move through the earth's
Marketplace
Today.
I do not want to touch any object in this world
Without my eyes testifying to the truth
That everything is
My Beloved.
Something has happened

To my understanding of existence
That now makes my heart always full of wonder
And kindness.
I do not
Want to step so quickly
Over this sacred place on God's body
That is right beneath your
Own foot
As I
Dance with
Precious life
Today.
– Hafiz

Chapter 29

Two months after two major operations. I still have cancer, but it's been remarkably reduced. The wounds are healing – liberal applications of vitamin E and rosa mosqueta oils are helping the scars. I can bend, move, walk, do chi kung. Even start clearing the garden a bit after two years' neglect. I get tired, and though I find it hard to be positive about that, I try to see it in the way that Jitindriya does, as time to stop, relax, witness what's happening. To sit in the September garden, watch the late flowers and the swallows.

Fear was often still there though. I only had to hear about someone's side effects from treatment, and I had them too. But I was also finding that, slowly, I was usually waking in the mornings with less anxiety in the pit of my stomach. Perhaps fear was something I needed to accept just as much as any other human experience.

> *Death is stripping away all that is not you. The secret of life is to 'die before you die' – and find that there is no death.*
> *– Eckhart Tolle*

One night I dreamt of a huge gathering of Tibetan Buddhists. There were so many of them that they seemed to form river deltas of maroons and golds as they moved towards each other.

I realised how many things had touched me since I had been ill that had Tibetan Buddhist connections. I recalled that at the end of a meditation a few months after I had been diagnosed I had suddenly found myself prostrated on the floor, 'seeing' a huge golden Buddha statue in an oriental temple, and just knowing I had once been doing this as a monk. There had been the 'chance' meeting with a Tibetan Buddhist monk and the visiting monks in Taunton.

More recently there had been Roshi Joan Halifax's *Being with*

Dying that had affected me deeply, then getting to know Jean and wanting to soak up her understandings and experience of the teachings. Now, *Grace and Grit* was adding to that, with its occasional mentions of how helpful Tibetan practices had been all through Treya's illness, her and Ken's relationship, and into and even beyond her death.

The chan meditation (Chinese, not Tibetan) also really opened something up for me. It helped me be a bit lighter, or maybe more open and expansive, about sitting meditation. I no longer felt I had to focus so rigidly on the breath, but could include whatever was happening much more. I could feel the effect in the rest of my life too. A greater acceptance, and curiosity about my experience right now.

This was exactly what Osho had been teaching, but it had taken me many years to even touch into what he was saying:

> *You are watching – then who is watching? Relax. In relaxation – when there is nothing to be watched and nobody as a watcher, when you are not divided into a duality – there arises a different quality of witnessing… it is just passive awareness… be non-tense, relaxed. Just be there. In that consciousness when you are simply there, sitting doing nothing, the spring comes and the grass grows by itself.*
> *– The Heart Sutra: Osho*

I had found tonglen practice increasingly helpful – breathing in difficult feelings, transforming them in the heart, breathing out expansiveness, clarity, freshness. Treya's words in *Grace and Grit* also inspired me in this. I learnt that tonglen could also be used to connect with others who are suffering, to breathe in the pain of cancer not just for myself, but for all others suffering from it. I came to see that it could help me develop more compassion for others, through feeling their pain, knowing we all feel the same things fundamentally, breathing it out for us all. This helped too in my relationship with Chetan. I realised how quick I could be to blame, and worked on seeing that blame and frustration, transforming that too. It's a powerful practice.

There was no discrepancy between Osho's teachings and those of Tibetan Buddhism. He had often spoken of Tibetan Buddhism's unique approach to death:

> *Only in Tibet have they developed the art of dying. While the whole world has been trying to develop the art of living, Tibet is the only country in the world which has developed the whole science and art of dying.*
> *– The Razor's Edge: Osho*

The dream about all the Tibetan Buddhists was encouraging me to go further down this path. And life was presenting me with the opportunities to do so. Chetan and I would go together on the Living up to Dying workshop, in a couple of months.

> I come to the end of a meditation in the garden. Two silvery wings flit in front of me, like a glimpse of a fairy.

Right now I'm on another medicine wheel workshop. I remember how in one workshop a few months ago I had just had to pick up the crystal skull that Carrie had brought, hold it in front of my face, stare it full in the eye-sockets, know it. I had cried plenty, but felt I'd absorbed its message, that one day I would go into death, there was no escape.

This time in the workshop I saw how I needed to get back in touch with the part of me that is thrilled to be in life, which delights, dances, knows all is well, lives exuberantly both in the spirit and in the body. The part of me that does know it's connected with the universe, but which wants to live in this body with joy, laughter and celebration. There was a 'magical child' in me which wanted to come out and play.

So it was perfect timing that the next day we were off to Spain for two weeks. Nigel and Judi had kindly lent us their villa beside the sea. Two holidays abroad in one year – when I was supposed to be dying!

The time in Spain was like a convalescence – for us both. As it was late September most of the tourists had headed off, but the Mediterranean was still enticing. I wondered if I dared walk into the sea, let alone swim. Maybe it would rip open my wounds. Or at least give me an infection. Could I do it?

Yes.

So good to have my feet in the soft sand, then to get into the gentle waves of the clear blue sea - and *swim!* Couldn't quite believe it, immersing all my scars in the water. A bit scary, but felt so good, so alive.

There was pain too, though mostly by now not physical – that just happened if I overdid things. If physical pain came, I was immediately scared I had ruptured something, which I had been warned about. I longed to be full of life and energy right away, but had to learn to be patient. It dawned on me that impatience was about *not* being present.

One night I dreamt I was being seduced by Rory Bremner! The dream was again about death. It was as though I would be fooled by this impersonator into wanting to die, which was often a strong force for me. I still sometimes wondered if it wouldn't be easier to die. In reality I could see so much in my life that was wonderful, and did not want to die yet.

This is my last chance to do writing, artwork, creative things - and it's important to do them. But even more important is the meditation, the opportunity for this that has been offered.

It was great to see Chetan having a restful time after all he had been through. Every evening we sat and watched the sun go down over the sea, while bats flitted around. In the past that would have been when I would have sat drinking a glass of wine, but now I hardly ever drank alcohol. My liver had enough to cope with. To my surprise, I found I didn't miss it, that I could just enjoy seeing others drink, and being there. One night a flock of hundreds of swallows danced against the crimson and gold sky. I could get drunk just on their exquisite dance.

We were quiet tourists, taking time to enjoy just being there. There were moments of feeling I was regaining some control of life through prayer and meditation, and feeling freer to move forward in my life.

> *I have just walked through the desert and have reached an oasis with refreshing water, a cool breeze and a hammock. I have reached a welcome refuge.*
> *– Daily Word*

Sitting outside the villa, overlooking the sea, and feeling well, those words are truly so. Yet I am also sad at times - for what I've gone through, what others have gone through with and for me, and for what lies ahead. Now I face death quite openly, even though I hope it is a long way off. I prepare for it, trying to be more meditative, to see death, when I can, as a great opportunity, a letting go. Of course, most of the time I don't see it like that, but as the loss of everything, and there is huge grief.

There was calm, too. If I paused, and listened, I could find guidance.

I thought of the swallows, gathering to fly down to Africa. Surely they are somehow guided. What a beautiful reminder they were of how we are all together in our journey.

One night in Spain I slept badly, with pain, and soon found myself in a state of anxiety. It made me look at the part of me that didn't want to be in a physical form, that found it too hard and wanted to just dance off into the cosmos. That part of me seemed like a little Tinker Bell fairy-like being. I told her that I needed her with me, so that I could live with the sense of energy and delight I had seen in the medicine wheel. I needed her dancing energy. I reassured her that it was safe to be in a physical body, and asked for help to hold this childlike energy, so that it knew the physical body to be a wonderful place too.

I knew this was part of my healing – to stop believing I could only really feel 'free' if I was no longer in a physical body, to know that being alive on earth is a wondrous thing.

> *Just be... and let things happen... Let the breeze pass, let the sunrays come, let life dance, and let death come and have its dance into you too.*
>
> *This is my meaning of sannyas: it is not something that you do, but when you drop all doing and you see the absurdity of doing. Who are you to do? You are just a wave in this ocean. One day you are, another day you will disappear; the ocean continues. Why should you be so worried? You come, you disappear. Meanwhile, for this small interval, you become so worried and tense, and you take all the burdens on your shoulder, and you carry rocks in your heart – for no reason at all.*
>
> *You are free at this very moment!*
>
> *– The Heart Sutra: Osho*

I was having the very occasional glimpse to 'let life dance, and let death come and have its dance in you too.' Surely life and death were always there anyway, dancing together.

Chapter 30

I was out of that glass box I'd felt myself to be in when I was on chemo. I felt connected with life again, though I knew there might be challenges ahead. There were.

I was due to have a scan soon after coming back from Spain, so that hung over me.

A new term had started at the printmaking workshop, and I was well enough to go, for the first time in over two years. I even drove there, an achievement in itself as I had barely driven at all since being diagnosed. Being back at the workshop was overwhelming. It was as though I was in another reality – in this familiar place, which I had known for years but where I thought I would never be again. And above all, my friends there. Hugs, joy, support in every way. I still had to be careful of heavy weights, but someone always offered to turn the huge wheel of the press for me. So normal, so extraordinary.

Fear of death is at times much less strong. Dare I say that? I know it can suddenly reach up and bite me again, but at other times I can feel so much more accepting of it, even sometimes welcoming of it as a great new adventure, a wonder and mystery which I wish to enter into as fully as possible when the time comes. But live, live, live first.

Sitting on the train before it departs, I watch Chetan on the platform. I'm going to London for the scan – he'll come up with me next week for the results. The train slowly pulls out, we wave to each other through the glass, and again I can't help but think of how one day we will have to say goodbye to each other more permanently. Or at least in these bodies.

After the scan I had some time before the train back to Devon. I went to Oxford Street, and found my excitement at being there hilarious. The shops, the clothes – how could I manage it all in time? So much for the great meditator! But this was life too, to be enjoyed. After two years of such illness I was literally back in the marketplace. I doubt if John Lewis ever had a more joyful customer for a new jumper.

Back home. A day of joy. I just felt happy, so very glad to be alive. Not for any particular reason, though it was a sunny, warm autumn day, blue sky, gold leaves. I spoke with my dear sister on the phone. We laughed. I visited Ali, drank tea and enjoyed her rumbustious kittens. Chet and I in the garden, him chopping wood, me clearing weeds that have grown so high since I've been unwell. Sharing tea and cake in the afternoon sun. Just a beautiful day. Thank you, God.

To London for the results. Shocked. There's new growth in the liver. It's in an area where there are lots of blood vessels, so it had been difficult to treat in the operation. But at least it's nowhere else, so there's no need for chemo. What a relief, but a horrid reminder. I try to move into gratitude – that I *can* be treated with an ablation.

Straight after the hospital appointment we travel to Chelmsford for an appointment to see Stephen Turoff, the psychic surgeon, again. It's perfect timing. We stay nearby overnight, and in the night when I'm feeling upset about the new diagnosis, I suddenly sense a tube of light or healing coming to me, calming and comforting as though someone is holding my hand. The session next day with Stephen is painful at times. He speaks about being in the moment, and as he works on my abdomen I am overwhelmed by love. I know that what happened in the night is connected with seeing him today.

Now when the bardo of dying dawns upon me,
I will abandon all grasping, yearning and attachment,
Enter undistracted into clear awareness of the teaching,

And eject my consciousness into the space of unborn Rigpa;
As I leave this compound body of flesh and blood
I will know it to be a transitory illusion.
– Padmasambhava

The ablation was scheduled for mid-November. Another November, my third since being diagnosed. I realised that it had taken a long time for me to take on board how far my life expectancy had shrunk. I'd had to do that at my own pace, not be told it full-frontal.

But the scan was a little way off. In the medicine wheel we celebrated Samhain, the end of the Celtic year. Letting go into the winter dreaming. We lit a bonfire, letting go of in my case rage, fear of illness, death… the usual! I committed myself to 'dreaming in' peace, to weave it into being.

There was great joy in just being alive. Yes, fear about the ablation was present too. But sometimes I just caught myself in a mundane activity, and realised how *extra*ordinary it was. To be alive. To celebrate another turn of the medicine wheel.

In the middle of London, alone, doing ok. Never thought I'd make it to this gallery, but here I am, one small person amongst thousands. Outside, the Thames flows quietly on past St Paul's.

Chapter 31

My new jumper is packed. I'm sure to need it in Ireland in November.

The small plane takes us from Plymouth to Cork. It feels like going on holiday, but there's apprehension too. What will it be like to do a course which is all about death and dying?

We drive to the Beara Peninsula, almost the most south-westerly point of Ireland. The landscape becomes more and more mountainous, with little inlets as we drive along the coast. By the time we arrive at Dzogchen Beara, which seems miles from anywhere, it's dark. Prayer flags are fluttering along the track that leads from what has by now become a small road, but it's hard to see much else now that rain has set in too.

Tumbling out of the car after the long journey, in the dark and rain, I've no idea where to find our accommodation. But almost immediately someone comes up and asks if they can help. We're soon settled into a cosy little cottage which we're told has views over the sea.

I wake in the night. The rain has stopped, the clouds have gone. Through our huge bedroom window I see a full moon high above a vast bay and mountainous headland, shining a path of light across the sea. I know I'm in the right place.

Daylight revealed a small group of buildings perched on the edge of Bantry Bay. We had a day to explore before the workshop started in the evening. There was a meditation room filled with Tibetan Buddhist imagery, its floor-to-ceiling windows framing the Atlantic Ocean. There are more prayer flags, a stupa, and rows of butter lamps outside the meditation or shrine room. Everyone we came across was so helpful and kind that it was impossible to feel like this was a strange new place. It was very special.

Perched even higher above the sea was the spiritual care centre, Dechen Shying, where the workshop would be held. I was curious about it, knowing only that it was a place where people with serious or terminal illnesses may come and stay. But surely that's not for me. Sounded a bit scary. Yet I loved the description of it as 'a place of respite in an environment of peace and outstanding natural beauty where people of all beliefs can come to rest, reflect and find meaning in life and hope in death.'

The workshop was packed with wisdom and learning. This was what I had been longing for – teachings that had been gathered over millennia about what happens as death approaches, and which honour it as a time of great importance in our lives, not something to feel ashamed of, a failure. I started to see how Tibetan Buddhism has given us in the West a great gift by sharing its teachings after its enforced exile from Tibet.

> *I believe the ancient Buddhist teachings on death and dying have a tremendous gift to offer to people of any faith or none, one that is offered in the spirit of Buddhism, quite freely and with no notion of conversion or exclusivity.*
> *– Sogyal Rinpoche*

It was a relief to be able to talk so openly about death, to listen to the teachings and to hear other people's experiences. We all resist change, but I was learning that to do so 'is as ridiculous as the river saying it doesn't want to flow.' 'Dying in this moment' – living with the possibility of death all the time – helps us to not be on automatic, to experience life *now*. 'The moment of death *is* now', Sogyal Rinpoche's words reminded us, and all is impermanent.

I saw more clearly the importance of letting go, not grasping. How else would it be possible to die without regret? I saw too the possibility of death as an opportunity for liberation, if it's possible to recognise that moment. There were teachings about what happens in the dying process – the dissolution of the body and the emotions, and moving into death itself. I learnt too a little about phowa, the practice for the moment of death.

I could see that a peaceful death could be a possibility. Two things, it was said, would make this possible: how we have lived our lives, and our state of mind at the time. Meditation, compassion and wisdom were the way to this.

Experiencing life *now* was fundamental. Because, of course, we are all dying in this very moment.

> We ride the crest of the Cornish waves, no longer just a joyful memory of something I thought I would never do again. I'm grinning from ear to ear as my board sweeps me back towards the shore.

There was talk too of practicalities – living wills, talking with relatives, what might happen to the body after death. Yet although this was all hugely profound, and at times very moving, it was uplifting and inspiring too, like the freshness of the wind and sea outside.

We were shown around the spiritual care centre, a stunning new building specially designed to give those who came the most special care. Each guest has a large bedroom facing the sea, beautifully designed to create a calm, caring, yet uplifting place. My reaction was similar to when we had gone to Sharpham, that this was a place honouring those facing death, providing the very best, not sidelining them. The people working there were of course the most essential ingredient in this.

> *I always think that each city needs a Death Centre. When somebody is dying and his death is very, very imminent he should be moved to the Death Centre. It should be a small temple where people who can go deep in meditation should sit around him, should help him to die, and should participate in his being when he disappears into nothing… And you will see the ultimate – the source and the goal, the beginning and the end.*
> – *The Heart Sutra: Osho*

We lit butter lamps, asking for prayers for ourselves and others. In just a week I would be in hospital for the ablation, but for now I wanted to be with what I had learnt. We had a day before we travelled back. The weather was awful again, but that felt like a blessing – we spent it quietly, going to the meditations, buying CDs and incense in the little shop, resting peacefully in our fogbound cottage.

The sun broke through briefly, and we drove the last few miles to the end of the peninsula. A rickety-looking cable car linked the mainland to a small island and announced 'only one cow at a time'. Steep mountains wrapped themselves round small inlets, and the road meandered through a village full of unexpectedly brightly coloured houses.

Strange that I haven't been able to write about the course. Maybe it's still being absorbed, and maybe I don't want to put the experience too much into words. Many much wiser beings have done that, and for me it's now about learning to live with those teachings. The teachings of impermanence, that all things change, and not grasping but letting go.

I really want to be more in meditation now, I can feel the effects of it - more peace, more acceptance, more being with what is.

Being at Dzogchen Beara has given me something beyond words. One evening I went into the shrine room by myself, meditated in front of the gold statue of the Buddha. It seemed so familiar to bow down before him. That devotional space. Yes, there's still fear and grief, but there is too a wider context of the flow of life and death, of them being continuous and not separate.

Back home, there was the ablation to face. This was my second one, but this time it would be with the NHS, at UCH, rather than in a private clinic in Harley Street. That first one had been painful for days afterwards, but to my surprise this one was much less so. When I came round from the anaesthetic I felt so lucky to have had it done, been given this opportunity. One of the biggest distresses was during the night I spent in hospital, when the woman in the next bed became extremely ill and crash teams came running. All I could do was pray for them all.

As we went into winter I was like a trainee tightrope walker. One moment I'd be balanced and confident, really getting the hang of staying on the wire. The next moment a big wobble, caused by fear and panic, would send me crashing. But I would always be helped up again. And I was becoming a little more confident in my ability to keep walking the wire.

I had to rest much more than I'd ever been used to, which wasn't an easy trick to learn either, as I'd feel fine while doing something only to be exhausted later.

Not a nice place to be, feeling knackered. But there's a lesson there, though one I find quite hard to learn - about pacing myself, and knowing and accepting my limitations, myself as I am now.

My next CT scan had been scheduled for early January before the ablation had been decided on. I hoped that as I'd only just had a scan as part of the ablation, the January one would be postponed. It wasn't. I watched as my mind instantly went into 'Oh god, they think it will flare up and spread really quickly,' then trying to catch that and look at it more positively. It was fantastic that they were monitoring me so closely.

I've woken up feeling good. Using a Tibetan healing meditation as I lay in bed, then the words 'It is my intention to heal' came to me. Part of me feels don't be so ridiculous, to set that up when it may come crashing down. But - why not go for that? It can only be of benefit to give my body that message - it's not denial, I know the score of how I am now and what may happen. But I can *intend* to heal, to be cancer-free.

Remember what Dorothy said: 'You can get through this.'

Talking with a friend who also had cancer, he spoke of what he planned to do in 2011. I was staggered at his confidence, to plan so far ahead. I realised I didn't dare look ahead more than a few days, or weeks at the most. I wondered if it was time to open up to things I might want to do in the more distant future. The danger lay in being disappointed – even devastated – if I couldn't do them, but wasn't it more life-affirming, juicier? And if I was worried about looking foolish if plans failed, I knew people I loved would only ever be supportive.

So what I'm saying is to open myself to the possibility that I may live a lot longer. To work on that assumption. To plan for it, so that I can do things I would like to do, be involved fully in life, available to life. That feels good.

I decided to apply for art college.

Chapter 32

There are dolphins in the bay, leaping high out of the sea. It's a couple of days after Christmas, and Chetan and I are in St Ives, watching crashing seas from a beachside café.

My third Christmas since I was diagnosed. I was full of joy, albeit mixed with twinges of loss for previous ones, fears for future ones. But I woke during Christmas night aware of something around my feet, and in the morning found that Chetan had placed a crackly stocking full of presents on the bed. For a moment I glimpsed the excitement and wonder of childhood Christmases.

> A sliver of bright orange harvest moon is ripening over Dartmoor. We're rich from the evening's dancing, laughing, gossiping. Old friends, new moon.

There was snow and blue sky on Christmas day, the snow a taste of things to come. Meanwhile there were tranquil days walking by an icy river, battling along the Cornish coast in headstrong winds, being together. And for the first time in my life, seeing dolphins. Magical days.

Sometimes there were nagging fears about whether I should be *doing* other things – changing my diet, trying the Gerson regime, having other sessions…

Yet amidst that I feel I'm also in a very different place. This illness has indeed changed me. I know and accept that one day I will die. There is fear there of course of the unknown, though sometimes too an excitement about what happens. Will it be an expansion, an extraordinary letting go into another realm of consciousness? I want to be available to that.

The hardest thing is the letting go - of this body, of the people I love, of my life here. It is hard not to feel sorrowful about that.

So, live fully now. I am so well now, even though I tire much more easily. Live, enjoy, deepen, be grateful, be loving, be expansive, be open.

I dreamt I was in an old-fashioned classroom where Sogyal Rinpoche was giving a lesson. Most of the other pupils were dozing or chatting, but I seemed to be incredibly attentive and eager. And indeed I did still feel very drawn to these teachings, and was finding the meditations very beneficial.

> *Doctors had told her the breast cancer was inoperable and would spread, limiting her physical abilities and causing death within six months. She refused to accept this. Instead, she decided to consider the disease a challenge. It gave her an opportunity: she could rid herself of useless goals and commitments and evolve new goals... make new friends, reshape her life consistent with the physical limitations imposed by her illness.*
>
> *She substituted the word* opportunity *for the word cancer, and there she was, ten years after the doctor had sentenced her to death, encouraging others to view illness not as a limiting affliction but as an opportunity.*
>
> *– Boundless Healing: Tulku Thondup*

Changing 'cancer' to 'opportunity' sounded a bit new-agey-positive-thinking, but I could see the value in it too. It was actually the opposite of denying the cancer. It was about accepting that life had presented this, along with many questions about what it is to live, to be, to die. I was grateful to still be alive and well enough to be able to explore them. Yes, living with cancer was sometimes excruciating, and at times I might have opted for a sudden death, but the truth was that I *had* been given this opportunity.

Another full moon shining in through our window. This time we're at Jonathan and Fran's, seeing in the New Year. So good to be here.

It had been an astonishing year. Being told I could have no more treatment, Mother dying, the operations, the ablations. Great extremes, a lot of learning. I hoped I might go into 2010 with hope, and start really seeing the illness as an opportunity.

What a good start to 2010. Sharing days of friendship, walking in the brisk air along the river as the sun was going down. The Somerset Levels quite flooded, the river absolutely flat and calm, reflections of the huge sun across all the waters.

Life is wonderful. Do I dare say that?

Yes, life was – is – wonderful, but little did I know of a challenge that lay not far ahead.

But the next challenge was just to get to London for the scan. There were massive snowfalls in southern England in early January. The snow was beautiful, and it was a joy to see Chetan tobogganing with our neighbours. But living in the middle of Dartmoor means that roads are often impassable, and I worried about not being able to get to the station. Not to mention what the scan might show.

The thought of being like this snow, melting away into nothingness, is hard. Yes, all changes form, returns to the ground, the river, the sea, but I find it hard to relate my being, my consciousness, to that.

I loved a bit in *Grace and Grit* where Treya talks of finding a point of 'passionate equilibrium'. That was how I wanted to live – loving life, accepting what is too. I determined not to let a bit of snow get me down!

I made it to London, where there was also lots of snow. Coming home was a challenge too. Even though the trains were running I wasn't sure if I'd be able to get back across the moor, but Chetan was waiting for me at the station. We saw no other vehicles apart from a snowplough as we drove back across the dark, snow-packed Dartmoor roads.

The snow melted enough within a couple of days for me to travel to Plymouth College of Art and Design to talk about applying for a course. If I did, I would just have to assume I'd be well enough to cope. I felt excited at the prospect, and determined to pursue it further.

On the night when you cross the street
from your shop and your house
to the cemetery,
you'll hear me hailing you from inside
the open grave, and you'll realise
how we've always been together.
I am the clear consciousness-core
of your being, the same in
ecstasy as in self-hating fatigue.
That night, when you escape the fear of snakebite
and all irritation with the ants, you'll hear
my familiar voice, see the candle being lit,
smell the incense, the surprise meal fixed
by the lover inside all your other lovers.
This heart-tumult is my signal
to you igniting in the tomb.
So don't fuss with the shroud
and the graveyard road dust.
Those get ripped open and washed away
in the music of our finally meeting.
And don't look for me in a human shape.
I am inside your looking. No room
for form with love this strong.
Beat the drum and let the poets speak.
This is a day of purification for those who

are already mature and initiated into what love is.
No need to wait until we die!
There's more to want here than money
and being famous and bites of roasted meat.
Now, what shall we call this new sort of gazing-house
that has opened in our town where people sit
quietly and pour out their glancing
like light, like answering?
– No Room for Form: Rumi

Back to London, for the results of the scan. Not good news. Although there is now very little cancer in the liver, there are nine tumours in the lungs.

This is not what I had expected, remotely.

There are nine tumours in the lungs, and although they're tiny they can't be ablated, as they're too small and too numerous. The only option is chemo, the same type as I originally had. I could either have it now or in three months as the tumours are slow-growing.

I had thought there might be more spread in the liver, but not this. For the first time I ask how long I might have to live, feeling I need this information to help me make decisions. Dr Bridgewater replies that I'm 'not average' – that I would only have been expected to live at most twenty-four months after the diagnosis, and it's now two and a half years. 'It's impossible to say,' he says. I like that, and am fine with the uncertainty, especially as it's on the right side of the statistics. It gives me confidence that I have generally done the right things, and can continue to do so.

I will have to make a decision about the chemo. To have, or not have. Now, or in three months.

We go back to Liz and Paul's, where we are staying the night, filled with sorrow. As we all sit together in a sad intimacy, my nephew Joe says that if he knew he was dying he would like to be 'as happy as possible without forcing it.' What a wonderful way of putting it, expressing the idea of equanimity. I hope I can live like that now, knowing the great gift of living and accepting too the great and necessary gift of death, when it comes.

In bed at Liz's. Outside I can see just a little snow on the ground. Mist is rising from the cold earth, and above it the sky is starting to turn blue and pink. It's very beautiful. Beside me Chet is sleeping. I feel so pained at what he is going through because of me. I just cannot put into words what he has done - does - for me. He is just absolutely there, accepting and loving me. Sometimes I feel so very sad about how my illness has affected his life, and that I may not be there one day to show him how much he is loved.

Chapter 33

Tumours in the lungs. Right from the start of my illness there had been a query about the lungs, from what was seen on scans. But now it seemed that there really was something going on there.

Dr Bridgewater had said that because the tumours were slow-growing I could either have chemo straight away or wait three months. I decided to wait – if I was going to have it. I would use that time to build myself up in every way possible – and to really enjoy those months, before the onslaught of chemo.

It was a painful time. Surely my death must be quite imminent. And I could only imagine what having tumours in the lungs must feel like as they grew – wouldn't it be very painful and distressing?

Thank goodness for painting, which was some outlet. And everyone I knew was so loving.

A meditation evening with sannyasin friends lifted me up, brought some peace and joy into the anguish. And there was the print workshop, where I was enjoying not just being back with old friends, but making prints again. The printmaking process provided a way of taming the wildness of my paintings, and gave me some sense of control.

> Ordinary life. Mowing the lawn on a dank August day, midges biting. Wonderful.

I had applied for art college before this new diagnosis, and when I was called for interview was unsure whether to take it any further. I decided to, and got in to a part-time fine art degree course. I just hoped it wasn't depriving anyone else of the chance, and that I would be able to cope. It felt like a fantastic opportunity, an exciting new venture – if I even survived long enough to start it.

So I must endeavour to live as well, as fully as possible. Not to go into terror at the slightest tickle in my chest. To enjoy this day, this moment. To believe that it is possible I can still live well and for a long time, whilst going further into my own being and connecting with spirit as I prepare for the day when inevitably I will leave the body.

Live well, live fully, live now. Hard when chemo lies ahead. But need to see that as a healing from the divine too.

As a Christmas present Chetan had arranged a session for me with a renowned psychic, near Eastbourne, in early February. Good timing. But before we left home I got incredibly anxious about finding somewhere to stay. I became distraught, hysterical, just beside myself. I knew it was about far more than accommodation. Chetan held me, soothed me.

I felt ashamed of myself, but did realise I was still in shock about the diagnosis. It was the whole thing of being ill, the latest diagnosis, facing death. And our friend Annie, who had helped me by 'guiding' the procedures in Germany, had died just a few days ago. Everything had built up.

The morning before the session we walked on the beach. I stomped along it. I was wrung out by my outburst, but still needed to rage a bit more.

I took great gasps of sea air into my poor lungs. The diagnosis has rocked me more than I'd realised. Perhaps made me feel it is pointless to still be alive, that the sooner it all ends the better. That's a painful place to be. Really, I want to live joyfully, consciously, in life.

The session with the psychic was good, though painful at times. It encouraged me to see death as part of life, not separate from it, and reinforced my 'life purpose' as to live more consciously. My rage was a good, creative force which could be used in writing and painting, and bringing death more into the open. There was interesting information about my work as an art therapist. Apparently I had worked in a temple in ancient Greece where art was used in healing, and in this life I had really needed to do so again, to show its potential.

A linen tablecloth is spread before me; a waiter brings peppermint tea in a silver teapot and sets it before me as though I'm royalty. We are in the Grand Hotel in Eastbourne. Chetan has solved the accommodation problem by bringing us to this treat of a place for a couple of nights after the session. If I'd felt like a helpless infant in my hysteria, this was just the place for that child to feel comforted. Sumptuous meals, attentive service, floating in a warm pool, even the bed turned down as though I am a small child. Which is, actually, how I feel. Chetan has provided this to comfort and love me.

We walked along the seafront, and along the pier. At dusk starlings whirled in a great swarm over the pier, moving as one.

Back at the hotel, wrapped in a bathrobe after a swim, I do a lovely Tibetan healing meditation I have learnt since going to Ireland. Breathing light into my cells, the light expanding out to other cells as I breathe out. Expansion, letting in the light.

> *With a clear mind, I can consider what to do next. I may choose to accept the help of the medical community. Or I may follow a different path. Whatever the choice, I remain aligned with a divine plan of health and renewal. I know and affirm that Spirit within is my health and strength.*
> *– Daily Word*

Slowly I adjusted to this new diagnosis. There was much to be grateful for. I felt well – no signs of anything in my chest. I was mobile. And I was often happy.

One day I walked up to Bellever Tor, where I had celebrated the end of chemo. I paused halfway up to look at the wonderful view. It was lovely, even in February, and for a moment I realised that instead of this leading to grief about what I might be about to lose, I just felt joy and intense gratitude. Something had opened up in me.

There *was* a growing sense of life and death not being separate.

I am. And always will be, eternally. Not the 'I' of the ego, but the 'I' of the timeless mind/consciousness beyond all personality, body, story. The 'I' of the universe that will, as Osho says, fall like a dewdrop into the river when I leave the body and join the great ocean of universal energy.

May I be at peace as I live and as I die.

I dream of my Native American guide. We're standing on a plateau, high up a mountainside. Spread below us is a vast landscape, which he tells me I have already travelled through in my life – despite my fears. I should be proud of the accomplishment, he tells me. Right now, on this plateau, I can rest a while, things are easy.

I'm aware that the mountain goes on up higher behind me, steep and craggy. There will be more hard climbing to do one day. But right now I can just enjoy being in this place, and know that my guide is always with me.

> *Individuation is an expression of that biological process – simple or complicated as the case may be – by which every living thing becomes what it is destined to become from the beginning.*
> *– Jung*

May I become all that I may become.

Liz and I hadn't been able to have our 'pampering break' in November because of the ablation. Now was the time. As we looked at what was available, I think we both started feeling that 'pampering' wasn't quite where it was at any more. We decided to go to Ireland, to Dechen Shying, the spiritual care centre. We would have almost a week there. I thought it was pretty brave of Liz, who had no idea of what to expect. But I put my worries aside, realising it was long past time for trying to protect her!

It was as special as the first time. We were greeted with a depth of care that was only matched by the beautiful surroundings. From my bed I could see the ocean, watch the full moon across the bay again, or the sun rising over the headland.

We went to the meditations, we walked, we talked and laughed a lot. We were offered time with the staff, to talk over what was happening. Chris, who had co-run the Living up to Death workshop, was wonderful. She made it possible for Liz and I to talk through some of the most painful, but necessary, things about my condition. About my dying, my death. About what I would want to happen as I approached death, what I wished to happen to my body, my funeral… Things like wanting to be as pain-free as possible, that I would like my body to be left for at least 24 hours so that my spirit could leave gradually and peacefully. That I would like whoever wished to, to accompany my body as it went into the cremation fire. Liz was so brave, so present, so loving.

A trip into the mountains eased the intensity. Our spirits soared as we travelled up a tiny road, high into the mountains overlooking vast stretches of coastline in the bright winter sunshine. We visited some ancient sites – an Ogham stone, and a stone connected with an Irish legend on which people still left offerings.

I like that feeling of being part of something very ancient. It reminds me that my life is short but also part of a great line of beings, still connected over time.

And I always felt very aware of Liz's love and care when I got tired. Thank you.

I spoke with Bronwen, the nurse at Dechen Shying, about my fears of pain and how it would be as these lung tumours developed. She was very reassuring, telling me about pain relief and discussing how I might be helped. It took a lot of fear away.

One of the special things about being there was that although we were completely cared for, there was a sense of it not being 'us' and 'them', as can be the case in medical situations. That we are all going through this together, this living, this dying, we're all exploring and experiencing it. We show each other the way; we travel together.

What lies beyond being in this body can surely only be journeying into greater depths, into light, into dynamic energy. I have seen it as darkness, but it cannot be.

I know I will be eased by my beloved fellow-travellers into that light.

I sit in the shrine room, meditating in front of the huge windows through which there is only ocean. A trick of the light makes the window opaque, except for the shape of my body reflected in it, which appears filled with the ripples of the calm but vibrant sea. That's exactly how I want to be.

Something in me has opened and expanded. It's as though there's more spaciousness in me. Perhaps more awareness of being in the moment without the grief of 'but for how much longer' coming in. I know that may not always be so, but I trust that it's something that has now opened in me, and to which I will be able to find my way back.

And so good to spend time with Liz. We had such joy, and such sharing. She was always just there for me, generous and open.

Coming home was good too. Seeing Chet at the airport, being back at the print workshop, feeling very fit. I could feel a change in me, an expansion that was gradually including death as part of life. Just as there is night and there is day, a natural and continuous change and flow.

Fear might arise. But so too might a simple delight like doing the shopping with Chetan.

Fear cripples consciousness, and fear is the source of unconsciousness, that is why without transcending fear no one can attain to full consciousness.

But what is fear? Fear is awareness of death without knowing what death is. Fear exists in the gap between you and your death, and if there is no gap, no space, then there is no fear.

Do not think of death as something outside you because it is not. And do not think of death as something in the future, because it is not. Death is within you, because death is the other side of life. Life cannot exist without death; they both belong to the same energy as positive and negative poles.

So do not identify yourself with life – because you are both. The identification with life creates the gap. And death has nothing to do with the future – it is always here and now. Every moment, it is. And when one ceases to regard it as something outside oneself and, so to speak, draws it into his consciousness and assimilates the idea of it, one is completely changed. He is in all truth born again. And then there is no fear because there is no gap.

– A Cup of Tea: Osho

Chapter 34

There was a month to go before the appointment to discuss chemo. Plenty of dread around, but good things too.

Our second wedding anniversary, celebrated very quietly. Chetan's birthday, spent in our caravan. We'd gone to our beloved Sennen again for a week, with winds so high we could hardly stand against them, but there was bright sunshine, eating chips on a glorious beach, and swallows making landfall as they arrived back from Africa. I found a place where I could sit high above the sea and meditate, like at Dzogchen Beara, though this time huddled in layers of windproof clothes. We walked miles along the clifftops and beach, and I was amazed at how well I felt. No coughs, pneumonia, pain, as I had expected to start happening.

It is as though my mind, my being have expanded by looking at the limitless sea at Dzogchen Beara, and it has allowed the space for me to include death in my view. And to see it as a continuum, life and death being intertwined, and 'dying' just the passage between two states of being, just as there is night and day, natural and continuous flow.

As the end of April approached I knew I had to decide whether I would accept having chemo. I thought I almost certainly would. The clarity had come in part from my session in Sussex, in which I had been told how important it was for me to learn to love being alive, to find joy in life. It seemed to me that I should use whatever means I could to extend that life.

Again I considered all the 'alternative' treatments – the Gerson diet, Oasis of Hope, natural chemo, eating cottage cheese and linseed oil… And again I ended up feeling that I needed the big guns of chemo, although of course supporting myself with all sorts of supplements and treatments. In particular, healing.

This life is so precious, there is so much to learn, experience, delight in. Having chemo says 'yes' to that again, to living as long and as well as possible even though it may be gruelling. To not have it feels like turning my back on life, giving way to a kind of depressive state of wishing life to end - which I think is different from accepting death when it does come.

We tried to find the rocks on Sennen beach we'd sat on when I'd sensed something wrong. Almost three years ago, but I was still alive. Yes, walking up the steep path from the beach was demanding, but I could still do it. Later as we lay in the caravan, listening to Sogyal Rinpoche, I felt very blessed – so normal, given so much and still experiencing such richness.

Back home. The scan and the appointment with Dr Bridgewater are in just a few days. I climb up to Bellever Tor, to mark my end-of-chemo walk there two years ago. I don't quite make it to the top, but get as far as the stone circles.

Walking into the first stone circle I know I am being held by the ancestors. This is a place where I can acknowledge my fear of next week. I ask to make contact with the 'spirit' of this cancer, and instantly see a figure made of fluid, transparent colours. When I ask her why this cancer is with me, I understand it is so that I come to see that life and death are completely intertwined; there is no difference or separation. I still have the cancer so that I stay on that kind of knife-edge, of knowing both life and death.

I tell the spirit that I now see that. I know that one day I will die, and that it will be part of a continuum, not a finality, but that right now I wish to stay in this miracle of being alive for as long as possible.

The cancer spirit seems to be sucked down into the dark hole beneath the burial stone at the centre of the circle. She really whooshes down there, and I pray that she will stay there, leave me.

The second circle. Approaching it I have a strong sense of

female love and solidarity, and inside it I'm surrounded by maternal warmth. It feels wonderful. I realise that this mothering is coming to me from many different sources. In this moment it is from the earth, the sky, the trees, the tor, the stones, and at other times from my friends and other people. I walk round the inside of the circle, touching each stone in gratitude.

Then to the big burial cairn. Here a sense of the warrior, of girding myself in preparation for the chemo. Of standing tall and proud. I know that Eagle Owl is with me, encouraging the warrior, the proud and dignified being in me.

A veil of early autumn mist in the valley, sun rising above it.
The land damp and fecund. Letting me live on it still.

Now, back home, the light is fading in the garden. The little fire I've lit is dying down. I hear the birds singing their last songs of the day, and I feel calm, warm, loved.

A few days later, the three months I had hoped to use so well came to an end. It was time for the scan. And I felt I had used them well; there could be no regret about having chosen to postpone the chemo, those three months had been so good.

To London tomorrow for the scan, but today a cream tea on the moor with friends. Sat outside in crisp April sun, long shadows on the fields, lambs bouncing around full of vitality, looking joyful to be alive. May I learn from that too!

Chapter 35

There was no cancer activity in the lungs. Nothing had changed since the scan in January. I did not need chemo.

I reeled out of the appointment which I had expected to take me into more horrendous chemo in a state of slight hysteria. And of course utter delight. I didn't quite understand what had happened. Had the person reading the January scan simply not compared it with earlier ones, which right from the start had shown marks or nodules on the lungs? Had there really been any change since then? This was unclear, and I was so overcome with delight that it seemed a little churlish to push the questioning any further.

What those nodules are has remained unclear. Maybe they're the result of a long-ago infection. No medical person has ever said they definitely aren't cancer, which would require a biopsy, but if they are cancerous they've been remarkably well behaved.

Unfortunately there was new activity in the liver, so another ablation would be needed.

But no chemo.

The future... anything can happen, I know, but perhaps there is rather more of it than I had been thinking recently.

Thank you, God, thank you, beings of light, Osho, spirits who have been with me. Thank you, all my loved ones, and all you wonderful, dedicated medical people.

I'm home. Coming through the front gate the cats run up the path ahead of me. The garden is lush, blossoming. I'm not coming back to chemo; tomorrow I don't have to go to the appointment in Plymouth to start it. I've come back to a whole new prospect in my life, to being well for a long time.

There was a certain amount of getting used to this new state. Like cracking open a carapace that had built around me. Slowly,

I could start stepping forward into a new part of my life. I was far from healed but feeling well. So many people don't have that in their lives; it was time to feel excited about life again, let go of the dread and grief. I even started jogging, very moderately, and really enjoyed feeling my muscles loosening and stretching.

A few days later, a celebration with old friends from Bristol Cancer Help Centre. It was almost as though I'd come full circle since that first Sunday after being diagnosed with cancer, when we had sat in the garden with some of them eating lunch and crying.

I dreamed a dream and I still dream of it,
and I will dream of it sometime again.
Everything repeats itself and everything will be reincarnated,
and my dreams will be your dreams.
There to one side of us, to one side of the world
wave after wave breaks on the shore:
there's a star on the wave, and a man and a bird,
reality and dreams and death – wave after wave.
Dates are irrelevant. I was. I am. I will be.
Life is a miracle of miracles and I kneel
before the miracle, alone like an orphan,
alone in the mirrors, enclosed in reflections,
seas and towns, shining brightly through the smoke;
a mother cries and takes her baby on her knee.
– I dreamed a dream: Arseny Tarkovsky

I started to see that although I had often found life very difficult, and had seen clearly my will to die, I also had a strong wish and intent to live. Paradoxically, but not unusually, I had found that through illness.

I also came to really *know* that one day I would indeed leave Chetan, and all those I love, at least in this life, through death. For a moment it felt all right. Natural, peaceful, not necessarily full of anguish. A completeness.

The distant sound of a tractor. Closer, a stream. Nearer still, rustling leaves, a bird singing above me in the tree. Then almost to my surprise the sound of my own breath. But of course. I'm part of the orchestra.

As the third ablation approaches I walk to the remains of a Bronze Age stone hut circle on the hill near us.

In the centre of the circle I bury a Dartmoor crystal, asking that bitterness, resentment, anger, and any negativity that has helped create this illness, be taken from me, and others. I call on the ancestors to help, and bury the beautiful, receptive crystal so that those energies can be absorbed and healed by Mother Earth.

It is early evening. In the distance a great streak of purple-blue where bluebells rise up from the riverbank. And I'm *here*.

The third ablation went well. They were not able to remove every trace of cancer in the liver, but I recovered really fast, perhaps helped by some new homeopathic remedies. Above all, I survived it. I don't think it's a risky procedure, but there was always that fear.

Back home. So good. Little things - opening a familiar cupboard, making tea, precious.

Even though yet another ablation might well lie ahead, it was time to relish my good health, my amazing fortune. I still got very tired at times, but was able to do so much more.

There were several family gatherings over summer, where I realised how much that net of relationships had held me. Some of my relatives had literally helped save my life, others I had not seen so much, but they were still part of that delicate weaving of love which had cradled me.

I knew that my illness had taken a huge toll on many people, and would probably continue to do so. I felt very sad about what they had had to bear. It made me also realise how self-absorbed

I had often been.

A couple of weeks after the scan I dreamt that I was being given the results of the scan – and the nurse was adamant that I was totally clear! Even though I knew that this wasn't so, I was amazed that my unconscious would dare to dream such an audacious dream. Perhaps the mind has to balance things, as a few days later I dreamt that I was relaxing in a deckchair when I was suddenly told by 'my death' standing behind my shoulder that I could die any moment, and felt that I would indeed do so.

So I guess that's how it is all the time - I might be well, I might die any minute. I know the message is to 'just' be in this moment now... I try! Now, sitting in the garden after breakfast, fantastic sunny day, midges still buzzing around. Bit like my mind!

> *To see through the eyes of the mountain eagle, the view of realisation, is to look down on a landscape in which the boundaries that we imagined existed between life and death shade into each other and dissolve… What is seen by the masters, then, seen directly and with total understanding, is that flowing movement and that unbroken wholeness. What we, in our ignorance, call 'life', and what we, in our ignorance, call 'death', are merely different aspects of that wholeness and that movement.*
> *– The Tibetan Book of Living and Dying: Sogyal Rinpoche*

As I moved towards the third anniversary of my diagnosis of cancer I seemed to be slowly creeping back into engagement with life. There were regular cream tea outings with Carrie, Ali, Shelagh and other friends. There was a ten-day retreat with Sogyal Rinpoche at Dzogchen Beara, taking me another step into these great teachings.

This time the remote Irish setting was filled with people, yet the atmosphere of calm and peace was only augmented by everyone's commitment and kindness. We stayed in the spiritual care centre, learning of other people's stories of coping with illness. Sogyal Rinpoche gave daily teachings, there was ongoing meditation, sharing good food, and those wonderful, spacious views which seem to echo the message of the teachings.

When we had booked to go on the retreat I didn't know its theme was to be healing through meditation. I learnt meditations that directly address healing of illness, but it was about something far deeper than physical healing too.

I heard one man talk of his illness, from which in fact he recovered, saying that he felt he had been guided during it.

I too feel that I have been guided. So much has been given and shown to me. I remember that time on the tube, about two months into chemo and going to see Stephen Turoff, when I suddenly saw that the woman sitting opposite me was holding a book titled in huge letters *The Power of Prayer*. It took a few minutes for me to even notice it, even though it was right in my face, and then for me to realise the message. Thank you, whoever you were.

While we were at Dzogchen Beara it was my birthday. I woke in the night with the realisation that I was 58 now. It felt solid, strong. In one of the meditations I saw a gift-wrapped box being held out to me. It was about daring to give a gift to myself, as writing on the box read 'May I be happy, may I be well' (words from Loving Kindness meditation). Perhaps I could allow myself to think – to hope, to dream – that maybe I could be well physically. I knew too that 'wellness' was much more than that, but could daring to see myself physically well be possible too?

Through the teachings and meditations I dropped more deeply into a place of calm and greater expansiveness. At times I doubted all that was being taught, only to realise the effect the teachings and meditations were having in me, and which I could see in the people there. It was a great learning.

Illness is not a curse. Illness is a blessing. It cleanses the mind.
– Sogyal Rinpoche

And that's what I think has happened. This horrible illness has cleansed something in me. Of course I wish I'd never had it, that I don't have it still, but there is blessing there too. I know I will die one day. I also know that something in me will never die. It never could.

Chapter 36

I never thought I would do this again. I'm body-boarding, being carried by the waves and grinning from ear to ear.

The Buddhist Loving Kindness meditation asks you to recall times when you felt really happy. Body-boarding always came to my mind, as well as sitting in front of Osho in the ashram in India. I truly thought my wave-riding days were over, but here I am. As for sitting in front of Osho – I think I understand a little more of what he was teaching us than I did then, and I am literally eternally grateful for being his sannyasin.

What I had been learning through Tibetan Buddhism was fusing with my experience as a sannyasin. They each seemed to cast light on the other, and I was in a place of far greater peace.

Another scan, another ablation needed. But at least there was no spread elsewhere. I had no idea whether the next ablation might render me 'cancer-free', and knew that anything could happen. Meanwhile, I started art college part-time, hoping my energy would cope with being a very mature and rather battered student, and finding it truly exciting. It was as though something in me had been released, and all sorts of crazy, enjoyable ideas for art were pouring out.

Fear and grief still come and go. I have a long way to travel yet in terms of acceptance and presence, but the glimmers of knowing that all is well, that nothing dies, sustain me.

That and love.

Chetan and I sit in a little café in Bude, eating jacket potatoes and watching holidaymakers braving the rain. It's three years today since I was diagnosed with cancer. We have some rather good homemade cake too. It's time to celebrate.

> *All the riches that you have can be lost, can be stolen,* will *be lost – one day death will come and will take everything away. When somebody has come to the inner diamond that is one's own being,*

death cannot take it away. Death is irrelevant to it. It cannot be lost.
– The Heart Sutra: Osho

And since…

It's a year since we sat in that little café.

I felt so well in that first term at art college – even driving, and coping with full days – that a scan in November really surprised me when it showed new tumours in the liver, and also the lungs. Unfortunately these were not amenable to ablation, so the only alternative was chemo. Knowing how well I'd responded previously, it seemed like the right option. If I did not have any treatment I would probably have had only a few more months to live.

The consultant also suggested one of the new, more 'targeted' drugs. If I lived in London there wouldn't have been a problem, but the post code lottery still exists and Devon wouldn't fund it. Eventually it was paid for through David Cameron's special fund. I got it thanks to the persistence of Chetan and my consultant, who fought valiantly with endless red tape. It was very stressful, but I was grateful to be having it.

As spring started to touch Dartmoor after a long, bitter winter, I was in the middle of chemo, struggling with blood counts, energy levels, blood transfusions… but still here.

I couldn't complete the planned cycles of chemo as I became unwell. My body had taken so much, it couldn't cope with much more. It was a difficult few months, with many reminders of the body's fragility and impermanence.

It's now four years since I was diagnosed with cancer. It is stable, but who knows what the next scan will show. But whatever that is, it will only show what's happening in my body, not my being.

When I can I walk by the river, remembering all the times it has received my fears and grief, and returned hope and acceptance to me. So much has been given to me, and while there is still pain I also know that peace, joy, awareness and just being are at the heart of everything. And, of course, love.

Death is not the enemy. It appears to be so because we cling too much to life. The fear of death arises out of the clinging. And because of this clinging we are unable to know what death is. Not only that, we are unable to know what life is too.

The man who is not able to know death will not be able to know life either because deep down they are two branches of the same tree.

Death cannot be the enemy. The whole existence is one. All is yours, it belongs to you and you belong to it. You are not strangers here.

Existence has given birth to you, existence has mothered you. So when you die, you simply go back to the original source to rest and to be born again.

– Zen the Path of Paradox #27: Osho

I am the Dance
And I still go on.

Afterword – Anand Chetan

A day or so after Diana wrote her final page of *Dancing with Cancer* she bled badly during the night. Dartmoor was heavily shrouded in low cloud and mist and the ambulance struggled to reach us. We were both unnaturally calm and practical while we waited. For me it wasn't until several weeks after her death that the real shock of that night surfaced. I remember clearing away the bloodstained mat and the washing-up bowl half full of jellified, clotted blood so that the female paramedic could use the loo. Then I followed the ambulance back to Plymouth.

Ten days later Diana recorded that night in her journal. It was:

'as though it was happening in two halves - the blood coming out, separating from the body, and the being, and whatever was left behind. Difficult to put into words.'

She drew two circles: one quite sunlike under which she wrote 'me' and the other, with the centre heavily pencilled in, described as 'blood and dark material, physical'.

'As I got better,' she wrote, 'there was at times a kind of blissfulness. I could just let everything go, there was nothing to do, just be.' Over the next few months the risk of serious bleeding was well controlled by regular endoscopies; a tiny camera went down her throat into the oesophagus and an attached gadget banded any distended blood vessels. We were very relieved to have the risk of sudden catastrophic bleeding much reduced and there was only one other, much less dramatic incident. Together with Liz we had a few days in a cottage on the west Cornish coast, past Zennor on the way to St Just. In mid-September sunshine, with a seal in the bay, we shared a very precious time. Once again Diana was able to visit Gwynver, where she had that ominous prescience related in Chapter 1, but this time it was a joyous day and she was able to manage the many steps down to the beach and the mile or so walk along the cliff to Sennen Cove with lunch at one of her very favourite places: 'The Beach' café that has views over a wondrous expanse of sky, sea and sand.

The stay was cut short with fear that Diana was bleeding again and we went to the A & E in Penzance. The doctor arranged for an ambulance trip up to Derriford in Plymouth. While we waited he gamely told us a joke: 'The situation in Greece is now so bad they are running out of both hummus and taramasalata… Yes, it looks like a double dip recession.' Liz and I packed up and followed.

It was a very difficult night at the hospital as Diana had made an 'advance directive', a 'living will' giving instructions that in an extreme situation she did not wish to be resuscitated. She really didn't want her heart restarted artificially or the risk of surviving but being severely incapacitated. We had discussed it with the GP and all seemed clear but it felt that night at Derriford that the directive, rather than Diana's current situation, was the staff's main preoccupation. While understandable, the medical team is legally bound to follow the patient's instructions, the only thing that mattered to us that night was treatment. If she had lost consciousness her own directive would have prevented basic care such as giving fluids to keep her hydrated. There was the possibility she might die from a bleed less serious than the one she had recovered from. We hadn't foreseen this and when we got home Diana withdrew the directive.

There was something else too. Osho says 'existence takes care very delicately' and her journal records a new receptivity to approaching death and an insight that dying may have its own harmony and rhythm that she could trust and be in tune with:

'The last bleed had an importance, a certain freeing from the body, a recognition of where I'm going perhaps. I felt the preciousness of life, but also a kind of lightness about it, that of course it isn't the end, and that one day it will be just a small and easy step into something else.'

That 'small and easy step' was explored in her dreams too.

'Dreamt I was probably about to get a new job, which I was happy about as I'd need some work into my 60's. Then realised I probably wouldn't still be alive.

Painful.

Then it was a celebration to mark the end of a course (possibly to do with the job training). Lots of us, first of all in a church or cathedral. I could see Dad there, and felt very happy he'd come. Then all of us 'graduates' went on to another little party, and I felt bad I hadn't been able to reach Dad, but knew he'd find me later, come and collect me. Before that all of us leavers were going on a short boat trip along the coast. It was beautiful and magical - dark blue sky and sea, twilight. It was a large cruise ship all lit up with bright, crystal-like lights. I knew Dad would be there when I got off it a bit further down the coast, and there was a sense of him, too, being very full of light.'

Diana comments, 'The dream was very joyful – and of course it must be about dying. It's reassuring and lovely, though of course makes me feel very sad too.' She shared it with Ines telling her that her father had been:

'glowing, illumined, at first just watching over me and then I knew he would be coming to meet me at the end of the journey.'

Ines felt that the presence of Diana's father symbolised 'the fathers' – the lamas and teachers. Diana found that very moving – and encouragement that her meditation was going deeper: 'A lot of the ngondro practice brings the root lama into your being – you and he become one, and he is indeed illumined. Take confidence from that.'

In a dream of Boxing Day 2011 though, 'the small and easy step' into death was more problematical:

'Dreamt I picked up a snake which had been around in my home for a long time - it was quite big, scary-looking, looking black and yellow, but I understood it wasn't poisonous, though was very wary of it.

I wanted to get it out of the house, it had been lurking there long enough. Picked it up with my hand over its head so it couldn't bite me. Was going to put it in the garden, but was afraid that if it was poisonous it might harm someone.

Then a long search for somewhere to put it began, during which most of the body of the snake dropped off, but it was still alive. I think by then it had bitten me - still not sure if it was poisonous - but I was more concerned with finding a place to put it where it wouldn't hurt anyone else. Kept finding field, gardens, allotments - was by now doing this with Chet - but nowhere felt safe enough to just leave it, so I was still just holding it tight and don't know if I did manage to let it go.'

Holding on to the snake, like maintaining her own hold on life, was increasingly difficult. Yet even while disintegrating in her grasp the snake could still bite. She'd like to put it down but there is no safe place. While this is mixed feelings about dying – fear and acceptance both – there is also something more: the wariness about the snake itself even though she understands, but only intermittently, that it isn't poisonous.

Diana was increasingly aware of an ambivalence to being fully on the earth – she touches on this when she describes the Tinker Bell part of herself. She didn't feel safe here, as in those lifetimes she recalled where she had been society's victim – or sacrifice. So while the tight grip on the snake is fear of dying there is also the wary reluctance to fully engage with living; to accept and merge with the snake and embody that unpredictable and dangerous potential for inflicting and receiving terrible hurt.

Normally she commented on her dreams as she recorded them. In this instance she simply followed it with a quote from

Osho that for her must have aptly summarised the dream's significance; the 'vaster Diana' is viewing a particular lifetime that was nearing completion:

> *The body does not contain you; in fact you contain the body. Ordinarily you think: 'I exist in the body.' It is absolutely wrong. The body exists in you; you are vaster, you are bigger – not only bigger than the body, you are bigger than the whole universe. It is awareness that holds all.*

The treatments continued. Diana was receiving Cetuximab at the RD&E but often the treatment was delayed because of low blood counts. Going there triggered difficult memories of her diagnosis and angry feelings about the way she had been written off from the beginning and refused access to surgery. Any hospital visit, too, focused her grief and pain at her situation and her anxiety levels rose as an appointment approached. She worked with this by visualising the RD&E as 'a healing temple' and 'a gateway into deeper healing'. Usually it helped but in mid-December the treatment was delayed for the third week in a row and we left the hospital and went straight to Croydon Hall, near Minehead, for a midwinter Osho Celebration. In the night she was very distressed:

'I guess I thought I was over it, didn't bother with the visualisation this time, and now here I am just so full of stuff that's almost beyond words. What's "the stuff"? That my body just isn't coping. I may die soon. Yet... it is dealing with so much, there's very little pain... grief, grief, hard to let go, to trust that dying is as ok as living. Jealous of people who aren't ill.'

She loved meeting old friends at the Celebration. She managed short walks, and amazingly, the 45 minutes of non-stop dancing in the Osho Nataraj meditation. The themes and preoccupations which are the fabric of the book stayed with her throughout the last months: her spiritual journey, grief, pain and rage at her condition, fear and a determination to pursue all options and live as long as she could. She knew it herself and at one point writes:

'The two things - joy and acceptance in life, and dread and fear, have to coexist it seems.'

Most moving and heart touching for me is her gratitude for life, even at its most stark and bleak. The journal entries often end with:

'truly blessed.'
'grateful for all I receive, for all I can give.'
'In bed now. Just thank you.'
'Thank you, beloveds in this life. Thank you, great teachers.'

Sometimes just a drawn heart with 'thank you' written around it.

On the 10th February she wrote:

'It's 4 and a half years to the day since I was diagnosed with colon cancer. Had Cetuximab treatment yesterday, staying in bed late today because it's really tiring me now... Today - had planned to have a little celebration, even aspirations of St Ives but much too tired. Perhaps just a small jaunt. But the main thing -

gratitude.

Remembering that, on a grey February day.

Gratitude to all who've helped me. Gratitude to life. And more and more gratitude to Osho - what a gift I have received from him - and to Rinpoche. Celebration in each moment.'

That fullness is there too as she records the preciousness of the ordinary:

'In bed, another gorgeous hot autumn day. Just now a sliver of new moon through the trees and an owl hooting loudly from the woods. It's been such a joy being in the garden all day with Chet – doing my practice, picking beans, darning, chatting with him...'

'Summer day. I've fed the cats, put the washing on. Such simple joys.'

One day in February Diana told me she dreamt Osho had been giving her sannyas. This was the initiation he gave us. Diana's sannyas had come by mail but for those of us fortunate enough to sit in front of him in India he wrote our new name, in Hindi and English, on a certificate, using a large fountain pen and drying the paper with a small oblong of blotting paper. Then he would add his beautiful and intricate signature, in Hindi script: 'with the blessings of Rajneesh.' For me it was the first time of being physically close to him and I was tense and nervous and my mind was racing. His movements though were utterly unhurried and total; he was doing absolutely nothing else but writing and blotting and this awareness gave his movements a grace and completeness. As he passed the blotting paper and pen to an assistant I could sense that total attention move to me. He leaned forward, placed the mala around my neck and touched the third eye. It was like being held in a beam of light.

This was absolutely a gift but also a gift on many levels. In Diana's dream Osho had been repeatedly placing the mala around her neck: 'He kept doing it,' she told me in the morning. Osho had spoken about the esoteric significance of initiation and when Diana told me of this dream I recalled some of what he had said. He had explained that in the past initiation was very difficult and a disciple may have waited many years, and waited without questioning, until a certain maturity and readiness was present in her being. In the modern world no one is ready to wait; the disease of the modern mind is hurry and Osho's solution was:

I must initiate you now and then prolong your waiting in many ways… then when you are ready, there will be a second initiation, which would have been the first in the old days but cannot be the first now.

The first initiation is a formal one; the second will be informal. It will be like a happening. You will not ask me for it; I will not give it to you. It will happen. In the innermost being it will happen. And you will know it when it happens.

Thirty-two years after she received the airmail letter with the Indian stamps addressed to Ma Prem Diana, the second initiation had happened as promised. It was momentous, significant, and frightening. It felt a preparation for death.

On the 18th February we enjoyed a lunch out with friends at the Riverford Field Kitchen. For me the days that followed marked the point where the real quality of life the surgery had given her came to an end. Bronchitis developed and she was very breathless and the fluid retention in her body increased alarmingly. On the 21st she wrote of a dream where she'd been driving her car, the yellow 2CV she'd had years previously, and other people had wanted to get in but they were messing about and dawdling. She was impatient; she had to be home by a certain time for a lesson she was going to have. The car started moving anyway; the brakes weren't working properly but it was only going slowly and was not dangerous. Only she had any awareness of what was happening – the others seemed wrapped up in trivia. She knew it was a dream about dying and must have seen reflected in the dream her hold on life slipping from her grasp. Her haste and sense of being pressed for time in the dream made her wonder: 'Is there a greater urgency than I had realised?'

A few days later she was dreadfully weak and sore. Yatro had told her: 'It's all about surrender now' and she hadn't liked that at all. 'Good to feel a bit of feisty fighting energy!' she wrote in response and then:

'The weather so lovely today - first day this year of really warm sunshine. Chet set me up in the garden, well wrapped up. Such a joy - blue sky, crocuses, warm sun, cats...'

She sketched the scene in the journal with herself on the lounger in hat and scarf, a cat nearby. She added a few comments to the drawing: 'feet up 'cos legs swollen.' 'Warmth and spring – enjoy, be in each moment' then the drawn heart and 'thank you'.

There followed a week on the crowded, hectic – hectic with dying – Cherrybrook cancer ward at the RD&E. Fluid was drained from her lungs and abdomen. Diana hated the place with passionate intensity. It is shameful that the dying are pushed into a side room off a busy main reception area with no respite from the stress and noise of the ward and their last moments visible to all through a window. 'Get me out of here' was her message but there was a new hesitant, uncertain, note too: 'I'm not good, Chet, I'm not good.' She was overjoyed when Liz collected her and brought her home.

On March 7th, just a week before she died, she made her final, and remarkable, journal entry. It was 'a horrid time, painful uncomfortable, the hospital pretty grim… the food really repellent.' She writes:

'Last night a rather wandery dream... but in each of the scenes there were lots of sannyasins.

We were about to do a meditation together. I knew I was ill, didn't know if others knew too. Felt very weak and unwell, sank to my knees and started sobbing. Was kneeling and crying into a piece of maroon silk cloth, which of course was about sannyas. To my amazement the sobbing gradually turned to laughter - hard to describe what I was laughing about, but to do with there being nothing to cry about.

Don't know if it was the same "scene" but then a group of us was preparing to learn a very ancient meditation - some very secret, arcane tantric one, based on all the energies coming into and out of the body. Not specifically sexual - encompassing far more than that. I was being shown ancient drawings and sculptures - probably Tibetan Bon - and knew that this knowledge had built up over many, many years and that I was privileged to be receiving it.'

She drew an image of a figure in meditation and another figure, inverted above, so with heads touching. The heads are drawn as though in sexual union with the fontanels depicted as male and female genitals – the seated figure receiving the male fontanel. Diana added her understanding of what she had been shown:

'The male and female had to become one, this was important. This happened by the fontanels of two of the sacred beings being placed together, and a tiny bit of the stone from the head of one of them entering the other. Could be sexual aspect, but felt it was more to do with what happens in phowa, the exchange of energies between student and teacher.'

Phowa is usually translated from Tibetan as 'transference of consciousness' and is the practice most closely associated with dying. The consciousness of the dying person is visualised as merging with the divine in whatever form is appropriate: the spiritual master, Buddha, Jesus or pure golden light. The practice can be performed for the dying person by a lama. In *The Tibetan Book of Living and Dying* Sogyal Rinpoche writes:

> *In some exceptional cases, the masters or practitioners have been so powerful that when they uttered the syllable that effects the transference, everyone in the room would faint, or a piece of bone would fly off the dead person's skull as the consciousness was propelled out with immense force.*

In the final stage of the dream

'we were all in a smallish room where we were going to do the meditation. Again wondered if the others knew how ill I was. Everyone sat down except for Maya, who had booked an adjoining side room from where she'd been able to rest whilst still being part of the meditation practice. She was quite mysterious - didn't look like her, with quite severe, pulled back hair, a darkish skin. She namasted as she moved backwards down some stairs to her room, almost gliding. Felt she very much wanted to maintain her contact with the rest of us.

Wrote this last bit at one the next morning. Have woken up with fear - what's happening? Especially that the abdominal swelling is possibly increasing, despite it being so soon since the treatment.

Not the best time of night to think of stuff like this.

Right now, relax, rest as much as possible. Let go, be in the now.'

There the journal ends, written in the early hours of Thursday 8th March.

Diana in meditation watches her physical form entering death – gliding backwards down stairs, the namaste both a greeting and a farewell. It is an extraordinary multilayered image as Diana had a close friend, Maya, who worked with the dying at Rowcroft Hospice. 'Maya' though is also in Hinduism and Buddhism the state of illusion. The soul, enmeshed in the body, sees the world as a projection, a mirage formed by karma and ego. This illusion conceals the ultimate Reality, Brahman, Truth. Sometimes the metaphor of the magician and his trick is used; we see the illusion only – and not the magician.

There is a further layer too because this concept is embodied as a deity in the Hindu pantheon. Maya is a Goddess, the Goddess of illusion, and Diana doesn't see her friend but a mysterious person 'severe, with darkish skin and pulled back hair'. When Diana felt the Maya figure 'very much wanted to maintain contact with the rest of us' it feels as if the dying part, that which had incarnated, still wanted to exist, maintain its individuality, its separateness, and persona.

On Monday, Gay, the hospice nurse, visited around lunchtime. It was clear that Diana's abdomen was once again filling with fluid and we discussed the options and whether further drainage would serve any purpose. Diana cut the discussion short. 'It seems,' she said to Gay, 'that you are saying I have reached the end of the road.' Gay was a bit taken aback, but had to agree. After she left Diana and I sat together, hugged and cried, and I felt her rather dazed by her new authority in taking charge of her own process. Her cousin Martin, the retired consultant who had advised so much in the early stages, and his wife Paddy, visited in the afternoon. There was much practical discussion about moving Diana's bed downstairs, commodes, and the prospect of Diana's next stage as invalid. There was a stoic and determined cheeriness but I felt Diana was already somewhere else. That evening for the first time as I helped her up the stairs she had to sit and rest halfway up.

She woke around 4am and was struggling to sit up. I ran round the end of the bed and helped lift her terribly swollen legs off the bed so she could sit up. She attempted to pummel the duvet with her fists and she said very distinctly: 'I am angry.' Then a long pause and again, very deliberately: 'I am so angry.'

They were the last coherent words she said to me. By 8am she was clearly dying. Ines came and began chanting: a beautiful gift to her dying friend that continued all day and the next. At one point Diana briefly rallied and with a radiant smile said: 'Ines!' and raised her arms. Ines just reached her as Diana's arms collapsed around her neck. Diana was peaceful, not restless. Yatro dropped by – and stayed. Liz arrived, then Nigel and Judi. Friends gathered.

Her breathing stopped the next afternoon. For a few moments I was with her in a cloudless clear blue sky. There was a tiny tornado of energy to my right, like a turbulent heat haze. Then I was back in the bedroom.

* * *

Diana had left meticulous instructions: what should happen if she died at home or in hospital, what should happen to her body and how her death should be celebrated. She didn't want her body in a drawer at the mortuary. She had been clear though that we should only do what felt comfortable.

> *I would like my body to be laid out somewhere at home, with my face visible, preferably for three days, and anyone who wishes to come, to come and be with the body. There could be meditation, music, whatever feels right, and the space made beautiful.*

The living room soon filled with flowers. We placed Diana's body on our massage table and Fred the cat curled up with her for long periods. Friends came, prayed, meditated, sat quietly with her, played music, danced gently. In death there was a strength in her face I had never seen before.

> *Maybe the body could be dressed in the dress I was married in – or the purple one. No make up! My mala and wedding ring to be on, and at some point the pages from Ngondro teachings to be with the body.*

About a year before Diana and I had discussed her wishes with Rupert and Claire from The Green Funeral Company and together with them we took care of the practical details.

In our death denying culture, but probably only for the last couple of generations, we have yielded up the bodies of our loved ones – and in doing so have failed them, and impoverished ourselves. Diana was following the Buddhist wisdom in wanting her body left undisturbed to allow her spirit three days to separate. Those three days were beautiful – painful and precious in equal measure and our grief had the focus of caring for and honouring her body. There is an unbearable vulnerability in the immediate grieving and the smallest detail can be everything there is. We moved her body with love and tenderness. We arranged the room to celebrate her and in deep respect for the mystery of death that we didn't understand. The next moment everything would be ordinary and normal – answering the door and preparing food.

> *I hope this is not too difficult for you all. You are doing me the biggest service and I thank you. Drink wine beside my body if you wish, have good music, eat good food, celebrate!*

On the second night after her death I went to bed around midnight. I became aware the room was full of love. This wasn't static; it was expanding outwards from nowhere, spreading through the room as though from an infinitely replenished centre. It continued for hours. There was nothing ghostly about it, nor was there any sense of Diana's personality or presence. It was simply love, but boundless, overwhelming.

Diana was definitely there though in the one dream I had that stayed with me. A few days after her Celebration I walked into a bookshop and in front of me was *The Illustrated Tibetan Book of the Dead*. Unlike all the other editions I'd seen this is not an academic tome but a practical, hands-on manual that restored the original purpose of the text: guidance to be read daily to the dead person for 49 days after their death. Much of the difficult Tibetan mythology is clearly explained or dispensed with. I was able to start reading it to Diana from day 12 onwards. It is the phowa practice and the person journeying in the bardo from death to rebirth is repeatedly urged to merge with the spiritual teacher and through them with 'the empty luminosity of reality'. At times there is a note of exasperation: 'It seems you still haven't understood so listen carefully… ' There are warnings about hallucinations, which must not become false paths, and guidance for different stages. As rebirth approaches, for instance, and visions show your future parents making love be careful not to be pulled in between them; don't be drawn into their sexuality and desire. Treat them reverentially as a god and goddess and perhaps you can avoid entering the womb again for another cycle of birth and death.

The night after completing the 49 days I dreamt I was in a stationary car in the middle lane of a motorway. There were others in the car and perhaps we were all dead. I got out and walked back seemingly into oncoming traffic and the next thing I knew was that I was in a typical Devon farmyard. Diana was walking toward me but her attention was on the stone outbuildings. There was no eye contact. She walked around behind me and became absorbed in a pile of farm implements. Suddenly there was a whoosh of energy up through my body and I said, or I heard: 'Go away!' Then a black screen rolled down and obscured everything – a bit like the theatre safety curtain in the interval. I was hurt and distressed; it felt contact with Diana had been tantalizingly close. Why on earth would I tell her to go away? With time I accepted that perhaps my grief was holding her back and my higher self needed to shock me into releasing her more fully. Perhaps she was lingering while the readings happened. Or possibly the 'Go away!' was directed at me: 'This is not your time and it is not right for you to be here.'

Diana's Celebration was in the village hall. As had happened at our wedding celebration our neighbours took care beautifully. There was an Osho satsang, the Hafiz poems that she loved, live music, family and friends. And a final surprise she would have enjoyed. The village hall has a stage and Ines and I whitewashed away the remains of last year's pantomime and displayed her paintings. They were hidden during the Celebration but as her coffin left, and to delighted gasps, the stage curtains were drawn to reveal the exhibition. Central to it was a series of six charcoal works: 'Days of my life' completed in the last months.

21,500: so many days, maybe not many more to come. As I marked the days of each decade of my life, unexpected patterns emerged. My life story, each precious day adding up to more than the sum of its parts.

With her remaining creative energy she sought form and meaning working with the basic components of her life – the days that she had lived. I think she had in mind the great naval memorial on Plymouth Hoe where the names of 23,000 lost seamen and Wrens are listed. She was fascinated by the contrast of that massive public edifice, exuding officialdom and authority, being also 'a repository for overwhelming, unspeakable feeling.' She relished the fact too that the monument is loved by skateboarders and a place where families eat ice cream and gaze out over Plymouth Sound. These are austere, rather formal works, exclusively in shades of black, white and grey, and are in significant contrast to the work which was displayed beside them and produced earlier in her illness. All those are in brilliant colour, ferocious and chaotic. Scrawled on the back are the dates she worked on the canvas and the feelings gripping her while she painted. One from Spring 2010 reads: 'How can I bear to have chemo? How can I bear not to?' 'Oh God what lies ahead? Run shout, scream, return to ocean.' And finally: 'Look for stillness.' We introduced the paintings with prose Diana offhandedly described as 'possible blurb for exhibition':

We jump into the water, swim, struggle, sometimes with luck just float. We hardly notice the far shore getting closer, until one day something grabs us by the ankle, tries to pull us under. Only then do we realise how deep are the depths, how fragile our bodies, how precious it is to be in those flowing waters. How much we do not want to be pulled under.

I was grabbed by a diagnosis of cancer in 2007. Though treated I was not expected to live long, but I am still swimming through those wonderful waters of life. They have threatened to engulf me several times, but many hands have helped me stay afloat.

These paintings have been part of staying afloat too – they're full of shouts, screams and tears, but occasionally and increasingly they also have moments of just floating that come rising like a benediction from those frightening depths. Perhaps they have helped tip that balance, and slowly blessing is taking over from fear.

* * *

For further information, and to view Diana's artwork, visit her website: *www.dancingwithcancer.co.uk*

Bibliography

We gratefully acknowledge the work of authors Diana has quoted.

Achterberg Jeanne. 'Transformational Journeys in Modern Medicine'

In *Shaman's Path: Healing, Personal Growth and Empowerment* edited by G Doore. Boston: Shambala 1988

Barks Coleman. (trans) *The Essential Rumi* Penguin 1995

Halifax Joan. *Being with Dying. Cultivating Compassion and Fearlessness in the Presence of Death.* Shambala Publications 2009

Ladinsky Daniel. (trans) *The Subject Tonight is Love. 60 Wild and Sweet Poems of Hafiz.* Penguin Compass 2003

Ladinsky Daniel. (trans) *The Gift. Poems of Hafiz.* Penguin Compass 1999

Maharaj Nisargadatta. *I am That* Chetana 2003

Osho. *A Cup of Tea* Rajneesh Foundation 1980

Osho. *The Heart Sutra* Element 1994

Paxton Dr Anne. *Opening the Door to the Worlds.* Basidian Publishers 2009

Rinpoche Sogyal. *The Tibetan Book of Living and Dying* Rider 2008

Thondup Tulku. *Boundless Healing* Shambala 2001

Wilber Ken. *Grace and Grit. Spirituality and Healing in the Life of Treya Killam Wilber* Shambala 2000

Woodman Marion. *Addiction to Perfection* Inter City Books 1982